HUMAN
HEART,
COSMIC
HEART

HUMAN HEART, COSMIC HEART

A Doctor's Quest *to* Understand, Treat, *and* Prevent Cardiovascular Disease

THOMAS COWAN, MD

Chelsea Green Publishing
White River Junction, Vermont

Project Manager: Angela Boyle
Developmental Editor: Brianne Goodspeed
Copy Editor: Deborah Heimann
Proofreader: Brianne Bardusch
Indexer: Linda Hallinger
Designer: Melissa Jacobson
Page Layout: Abrah Griggs

Printed in the United States of America.
First printing October, 2016.
10 9 8 7 6 5 4 3 2 1   16 17 18 19 20

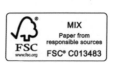

g green press INITIATIVE

Chelsea Green Publishing is committed to preserving
ancient forests and natural resources. We elected to print
this title on 100-percent postconsumer recycled paper,
processed chlorine-free. As a result, for this printing, we
have saved:

63 Trees (40' tall and 6-8" diameter)
29 Million BTUs of Total Energy
5,444 Pounds of Greenhouse Gases
29,527 Gallons of Wastewater
1,976 Pounds of Solid Waste

Chelsea Green Publishing made this paper choice because
we and our printer, Thomson-Shore, Inc., are members
of the Green Press Initiative, a nonprofit program
dedicated to supporting authors, publishers, and suppliers
in their efforts to reduce their use of fiber obtained
from endangered forests. For more information, visit:
www.greenpressinitiative.org.

Environmental impact estimates were made using the Environmental Defense Paper Calculator.
For more information visit: www.papercalculator.org.

Our Commitment to Green Publishing

Chelsea Green sees publishing as a tool for cultural change and ecological stewardship.
We strive to align our book manufacturing practices with our editorial mission and to
reduce the impact of our business enterprise in the environment. We print our books
and catalogs on chlorine-free recycled paper, using vegetable-based inks whenever possible. This book may cost slightly more because it was printed on paper that contains
recycled fiber, and we hope you'll agree that it's worth it. Chelsea Green is a member of
the Green Press Initiative (www.greenpressinitiative.org), a nonprofit coalition of publishers, manufacturers, and authors working to protect the world's endangered forests
and conserve natural resources. *Human Heart, Cosmic Heart* was printed on paper supplied by Thomson-Shore that contains 100% postconsumer recycled fiber.

Library of Congress Cataloging-in-Publication Data
Names: Cowan, Thomas, 1956- author.
Title: Human heart, cosmic heart : a doctor's quest to understand, treat, and prevent
    cardiovascular disease / Thomas Cowan.
Description: White River Junction, Vermont : Chelsea Green Publishing, [2016] |
    Includes index.
Identifiers: LCCN 2016026012| ISBN 9781603586191 (pbk.) | ISBN
    9781603586207 (ebook)
Subjects: | MESH: Cardiology | Heart Diseases | Philosophy, Medical | Personal
    Narratives
Classification: LCC RC685.C6 | NLM WG 21 | DDC 616.1/2--dc23
LC record available at https://lccn.loc.gov/201602601

Chelsea Green Publishing
85 North Main Street, Suite 120
White River Junction, VT 05001
(802) 295-6300
www.chelseagreen.com

MIX
Paper from
responsible sources
FSC® C013483

"People may say I am crazy. Perhaps they are right. In this case, it is not so much important if there is one fool more or less in the world. But in case that I am right and science is wrong, Lord have mercy on Mankind."

—VIKTOR SCHAUBERGER

"Tears come from the heart and not from the brain."

—LEONARDO DA VINCI

CONTENTS

CHAPTER ONE

Doubting Thomas

I can see myself at sixteen years old, exhausted and slumped on the locker room bench. My teammates have long since showered and gone home. Eventually Coach Callaway sticks his head in and barks, "Can't take all day, Cowan! Have to lock up here."

I'm not scared, just curious.

With intense basketball practice five days a week, I can't figure out why I never get into shape. Our team was ranked among Michigan's top ten, even against the urban schools that regularly sent players to top colleges or occasionally the NBA, and our practices were grueling. Coach Callaway, whose ambitions lay beyond high school coaching, made us run laps if I failed to sink ten consecutive foul shots. Our style, and our strategy, was to run the other team into the ground.

And yet, even long after we finished practice, my heart races—jumping suddenly from 72 beats per minute to 200—and I can't do anything about it except wait for it to pass. I never tell anyone, embarrassed about my poor conditioning and worried that I will lose valuable playing time if I let on how tired I feel. Once it calms down, I trudge home through the dark to our house in suburban Detroit.

———◆———

My earliest clear memory is of hiding in my bedroom closet furious with the world and yet hoping someone (mostly my mother) would come, offer a kind word, and rescue me from my misery. I don't remember what provoked this particular episode, but I do remember that it happened somewhat frequently and that, even from an early age, I liked to play alone and rarely took up the chance to play with other children. I rarely spoke, and when I did, it was with a terrible stutter and speech impediment that prevented me from pronouncing my *L*'s.

When I was six, my worried parents took me to a child psychiatrist, who told them that I just thought a lot and that someday I might decide to share what I was thinking. There were no more visits, there was no therapy, no intervention at all—something I've remained profoundly grateful for to this day, especially during patient visits with young children and their concerned parents.

I did have speech therapy at school to correct the impediment, and I stopped stuttering around the time I was seven. My speech teacher commented that I was the only student she had had who successfully, and totally, corrected a speech impediment. It was because, if there was one thing I was good at, it was practicing things to perfection, especially things I could do myself that didn't require me to participate with others. I spent hours in front of the mirror making my tongue do the right movement as I repeated words that began with *L*.

In this same way, I practiced *ad infinitum* every other physical skill I was exposed to. By age three, I could catch a ball as high as my father could throw it. Later, I set up a basketball court in my bedroom, wearing the rug down to the wood underneath. I practiced golf for hours, shot hockey pucks into a shoe box for hours, and threw rubber balls against the side of our house into the painted strike zone on the wall for hours—always by myself and always working on perfecting technique and form. Even as a six-year-old, I could not tolerate a hitch in my throw or improper footwork on a reverse layup. If I couldn't do it, I practiced it until I could. My form and appearance had to be perfect. I needed to master whatever I set my mind to, to take things to their logical conclusions.

This drive for mastery collided with a skepticism that often comes naturally to kids before adulthood outfits us with blinders. As I was memorizing the order of the US presidents backward and forward and reading every story I could about Native peoples and how they lived, I couldn't make sense in my mind of the way American history had unfolded, driven as it so often was, and is, by greed over money, land, possessions, and power—all in the context of liberty and justice for all. And I remember trying to understand, really understand, what the big deal was about gold. I liked food, and I was practical about money, so I didn't get why people cared so much about gold, which you can't even eat, and seemed to have no inherent value, at least that I could fathom. Plenty of things resist degradation and could be used for trade. Why gold? It came early to me that adult explanations often make no sense.

Sometimes teachers called me Doubting Thomas because I had such a hard time accepting authority figures or teachers, especially if the answer to "Why?" was "Because someone said so." But I learned to live in contradictory worlds, to a certain extent, although the contradictions never escaped me. My father and grandfather were dentists, and it was clear to me, although I hated the idea of it, that I was meant to become a doctor. One day, my father had me spend a day with one of his doctor friends—"This is Tommy. He wants to be a doctor one day."—when an obese African American patient came in complaining of a chronic cough she couldn't get to go away.

"Dr. Klein, why won't my cough go away?" she asked, as I stood nearby listening.

"It's the bad air in Detroit," he replied.

"Then why don't you cough?" she replied.

I burst out laughing and was not invited back.

Racial tensions in Detroit at the time were high. Twenty percent of the students at our suburban school were African Americans who were bussed in from the housing projects. Most of the rest of us were Jewish. The Jewish and the African American students had little to do with each other, took no classes together, never socialized together, and usually only met in conflict. But I was one of the stars on an otherwise all black and very successful basketball team. I was grudgingly accepted, if never embraced, because I had some useful skills—mainly a perfect jump shot—although I always struggled with the social environment on the team. I was nicknamed The Professor, but I could shoot, so I stuck.

———◆———

In the summers, my parents sent me off to camp, which I hated because the counselors forced me to participate in group activities instead of leaving me alone to do what I wanted. But every year, there was a week-long canoe trip in the wilderness of Algonquin Provincial Park in northern Ontario, a paradise of more than a thousand miles of interconnected canoe routes. This canoe trip gave me a feeling I loved that I could never recreate during everyday life in suburban Detroit. I was so happy and so at peace that I could ignore being in such close contact with other people day in and day out.

When I was seventeen, my sister, a few friends, and I set out for a week-long canoe trip on our own in Algonquin Provincial Park. It was magical. The peace, the sense of freedom, even developing relationships and deeper connections with the other people on the trip was like nothing I'd ever experienced.

On the last night of our trip, as we floated in the middle of a lake whose name I have long since forgotten, we were treated to an hour-long performance of the northern lights. The northern lights are magical for everyone who experiences them, but it was particularly sensational for us because we had no idea such a thing existed. The final day of our trip and the drive home was spent wondering and talking about God and our mystical experience.

Those lights let me experience awe and feel for the first time that I was somehow related to the wider cosmos. I felt as though I'd put my finger on the pulse of something real. I knew, from the deepest part of my being, from the heart, that I was experiencing something true and extremely powerful.

For my entire life, I have been in awe of the heart, both in the medical, physical, and anatomical sense and in the broader, spiritual, and sacred sense. It has presented me with the only significant personal medical condition I've ever confronted, and it has also presented me with the most important insights I've ever had about what it means to love and connect in an authentic way with other human beings and with the world. It has offered me challenges—physical and intellectual—as I've struggled to understand what it really does in the body, as well as a compass for my personal and professional journey as a doctor. As a young boy first facing out toward the world, as a young doctor first setting out in it to help people heal and recover, and now as an older man, husband, and grandfather looking back on a life and the threads that run through it, I see my heart, the human heart, the cosmic heart at the center of it.

In looking back at my life, and looking forward to the world of my grandchildren, I know that the heart can be a source of disease—and is for far too many people—but that it can also be a wellspring of health. We need to strive for a deeper, more accurate understanding of what makes the heart tick. We need to reexamine how the blood circulates in the body, and revise our understanding of why and how the heart gets sick and how to heal an ailing heart. And we need to do this in the context of society and its injustices, and our ecosystems and the damage we've done to them, in much the same way we must treat the heart, not in isolation, but within the context of the body.

CHAPTER TWO

Circulation

I n 1628, an English physician named William Harvey published what would become a seminal work in the field of
cardiology, a book titled *Exercitatio Anatomica de Motu
Cordis et Sanguinis in Animalibus* (*Anatomical Studies on the
Motion of the Heart and Blood in Animals*), often referred to
simply as *De Motu Cordis*. At the time it was published—at the
crux of Europe's scientific revolution—*De Motu Cordis* was met
with both praise and opposition. Today, Harvey is considered
one of the most important scientists and physicians of all time
for his study of circulation, his description of the heart as a
pump, his empirical methodology—and for dealing a deathblow
to the theory of vitalism.

Until Harvey published *De Motu Cordis*, it was the Greek
physician Galen's view of circulation that prevailed. Galen's theory was that the liver was the origin of venous blood and that
blood and spirits flowed from the heart in the arterial system.
Dr. Harvey, who served as physician to King James I, King

Charles I, and Sir Francis Bacon and would later in his career defend women against allegations of witchcraft, rejected the idea of a vital force as the engine for the movement of blood around the body. Today, most scientists continue to reject any suggestion of an unseen force playing a role in how things work. Harvey's description of the heart as a pump remains one of the most important foundations of modern medicine and physiology.

I was already disillusioned with the modern worldview—the dominant paradigm, industrial capitalism, whatever you want to call it—when I first encountered Rudolf Steiner's idea that the three most important "things" for the further evolution of humanity are: (1) that people stop working for money, (2) that people realize there is no difference between sensory and motor nerves, and (3) that the heart is not a pump.

Because I was already skeptical of so much, encountering these ideas—and, by extension, Steiner's worldview—wasn't the gut-wrenching struggle for me that it is for some people. I was surprised but not incredulous to encounter Steiner's way of thinking and viewing the world. More than anything, it felt like coming home. Like something I knew all along but had never seen articulated.

The idea of Steiner's that interested me the most was that the heart is not a pump. It was an idea that would continue to intrigue me for decades and drove me to question everything I'd learned about the heart and circulation. By *circulation*, I mean the movement of blood in the blood vessels, of which there are basically three types: arteries, veins, and capillaries. When blood exits the heart, it travels through the large aortic arch into the major arteries and then into the small arterioles until it meets the "midpoint," that is, the capillaries.

Capillaries are the one-layer thick transition vessels where nutrients and gases are exchanged between the blood and the cells. The capillary system is massive; if it were spread out, it would cover at least one entire football field.[1] After the blood exits the capillaries, it enters the smallest venules in its trip back to the heart. From the small venules, it goes to the progressively larger veins and then finally into the largest veins like the inferior and superior vena cava that bring all of the blood back from the body to the heart and lungs. The purpose of this circulation is to bring oxygenated, nutrient-rich blood to the cells where it is needed and then bring the oxygen-poor, nutrient-poor blood back to the heart and lungs so that it can be replenished.

There are profound mysteries in even this simple description of circulation. Although they aren't etymologically connected, the words *arteries* (ars, or Mars) and *veins* (Venus) suggest a cosmic or not-of-the-earth connection. And the heart—which people have, for millennia, associated with the sun—lies between these archetypal male and female principles. Each half of the circulation has an archetypal disease pattern: The arteries are the location where hypertension, a predominantly male disease, plays out. The veins are prone to varicose veins, a predominantly female disease.

If you examine the relative velocity of the blood at various stages of the circulation, you'll see that the blood moves the fastest in the large arteries and veins, where it is forced into comparatively fewer channels, and the blood moves the slowest in the capillaries, because there are so many of them. This is similar to how water moves in a river. It is fastest when the river is narrow, slower when it flows out into tributaries, and slowest when it flows out into a wetland area.

What's amazing is that blood actually stops moving in the capillaries, which is necessary for the efficient exchange of gases, nutrients, and waste products. After the blood stops moving, it oscillates slightly, and then begins to flow again as it enters the veins. But if the blood stops moving at the midpoint of its circular flow through blood vessels, only then to start moving again, what is the force that drives this movement of the blood from its motionless state before it leaves the capillaries and begins its journey back to the heart? Is it possible that this force is the "pumping" of the heart? Wouldn't there have to be some pump located in the capillaries propelling the blood forward and upward? Is there some "vital" force located in the capillaries that does this pumping? These are the questions we must grapple with if we're going to understand how the blood circulates in the body. But one thing is clear: If the blood has stopped moving inside the capillaries, then the force cannot come from the heart. It must arise in the capillaries.

In order to understand that precise moment in the capillaries when the blood begins to move again, it's worth examining the nature of water, which offers critical insight into an understanding of how and why the blood moves. We are taught in science class that matter exists in three states: solid, liquid, and gas. Every substance, depending on the conditions, exists in one of these states, and these are all the possible states that exist. If you think of water, however, you realize that it exhibits properties that seem to defy this three-state model—a model that provides one of the bedrock principles of modern science. We learn that as a substance moves from gas to liquid to solid, the molecules get closer together and the substance becomes denser. As a result, the volume of a given liquid substance is heavier than an equivalent volume of the same substance in its gaseous state, and the solid is denser and heavier still than the liquid. For example, liquid mercury is heavier than gaseous mercury, and solid mercury sinks in liquid mercury because it is denser and heavier. But this is not the case for water. Only with water does the solid phase (ice) float on the liquid phase (water). If solid water were heavier than liquid water, aquatic life as we know it could not exist.

We have all witnessed surface tension, which is the surprising and unusual tendency of the top layer of a body of water to be extremely "thick" or "strong." Most scientific explanations say that this is because the interface between the air and the water produces a force that changes the molecular configuration of the topmost three or four molecular layers of water so that it becomes "more dense." But can we really water-ski or skip heavy rocks across a three- or four-molecular thick "layer" of water? That's the thickness of the closest together you can hold your thumb and index finger divided by a million. And even if it is true, what is meant by the changed molecular configuration of this dense water? Is it water or not? If it's a different molecular configuration than water, what do we call it?

Dr. Gerald Pollack is a researcher and professor of bioengineering at the University of Washington who has been investigating the anomalous behaviors of water and the so-called fourth phase for many years. Viktor Schauberger was an Austrian forester, inventor, and intellectual who died in 1958. If you study the work of Pollack and Schauberger together, it offers some startling insights into the behavior of water.

Pollack has found that water exists in not three but four "phases." The fourth phase is an intermediary between liquid, or bulk, water and the solid phase of ice. There have been many names given to this fourth phase. Pollack calls it the exclusion zone or exclusion layer, but other names include the colloidal phase, gel phase, or structured water. I refer to it as structured water because for me the most important aspect of this anomalous phase is that it is more structured than bulk water.

Pollack describes in his book, *The Fourth Phase of Water*, how structured water forms. Any time you have a hydrophilic surface such as gelatin or nafion (a plastic) and you put it in water, a zone of structured water will form. The thickness depends on the charge on the surface of the hydrophilic substance and some other factors, which I will explain in greater detail in chapter 7.

This ability of a hydrophilic substance to convert bulk water into structured water explains why, when you put strongly hydrophilic proteins like gelatin in water under the proper conditions, you create a solid "gel" of structured water. This is how

Exclusion Zone (EZ)

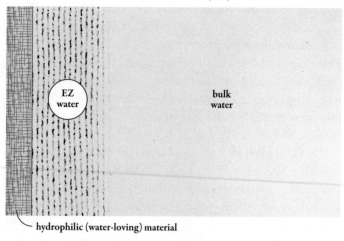

hydrophilic (water-loving) material

Any time you put a hydrophilic surface—such as gelatin or nafion (a plastic)—in water, a zone of structured water will form. This zone is sometimes referred to as the exclusion zone (EZ) because it excludes toxins, solutes, and other substances. Reproduced with permission from Gerald H. Pollack, The Fourth Phase of Water *(Washington, DC: Ebner and Sons Publishers, 2013), xxii.*

you make Jello, which can give us some insight into some of the properties of this fourth phase. This fourth phase of water forms best at certain temperatures (around 4°C),[2] and it highly structures the bulk water, which is why Jello doesn't leak (unless you heat it and convert it back to water) even though it's more than 96 percent water by volume.

This ability of highly hydrophilic substances, especially proteins, to structure water is central to biological life. The majority of the water in biological systems, including in cells, is in the form of structured water. This is why our cells, like Jello, don't leak even though our cells are about 70 percent water. The cytoplasm in our cells is in a gel-like state because of the network of hydrophilic proteins that make up the interior framework of the cell.

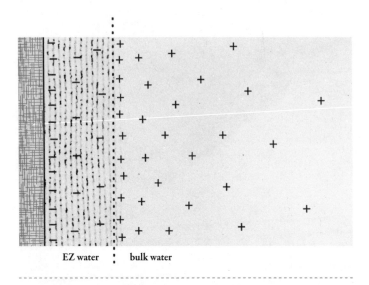

EZ water ⋮ bulk water

As water becomes structured, the electrical charges separate. The structured water becomes negatively charged while the bulk water is positively charged. Reprinted by permission from Pollack, 82.

There are many interesting properties of the structured water that forms right next to these hydrophilic surfaces. These include having an increased viscosity compared to bulk water. The structured water layer is also negatively charged as a result of having an abundance of free electrons. The presence of these free electrons is an intrinsic part of the structuring process of water. As the water becomes structured, it also becomes negatively charged. This can be shown by placing a voltage meter in the structured zone and comparing the measurement to a voltage meter placed in the bulk water zone.[3]

Another property of structured water is that the pH of the structured water zone is different from that of the bulk water, which can also be confirmed by careful pH measurements.[4] There are also other physical differences between structured water and bulk water. The molecular configuration of the

Nafion tube filled with water

(a)

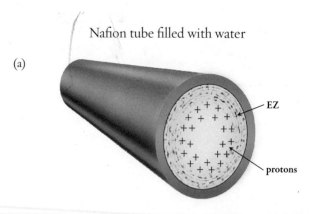

(b)

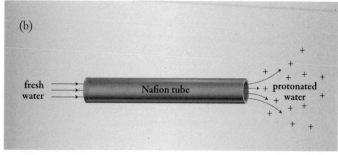

A hydrophilic tube with a layer of structured water lining the inside of the tube. Reprinted by permission from Pollack, 75.

structured water zone is more dense than that of bulk water. Most important, however, is that, simply as a result of a hydrophilic surface being placed in bulk water, with essentially no outside inputs, a layer of structured water forms next to the hydrophilic surface that has a different chemical (pH), electrical (voltage), and molecular configuration (density) than bulk water. This is a dramatic revelation in and of itself.

The next step—and the one crucial to understanding circulation—is that if you take the hydrophilic surface and roll it up into a tube, you produce a hydrophilic tube with a layer of structured water lining the inside of the tube. Again, this is with no outside input; it's simply a result of the interaction between the hydrophilic surfaces and bulk water. Then, within this tube, something astounding happens. As a result of the separation of electrical charges—again, the natural and inevitable consequence of the interaction of a hydrophilic tube and water—the bulk water will begin to flow from one end of the tube to the other and then out. Furthermore, this flow will be indefinite, unless acted upon by a force that stops it.

This is hugely significant because it means that all you need to do to get water to flow, and for mechanical work to be done, and for it to be done indefinitely, is to put a hydrophilic tube in a pot of water.

This is a perpetual motion machine! How can this be? Where does the separation of charges (i.e., the voltage) come from? This has huge repercussions for the way one can generate "work," which is a consequence of flow or movement. Currently, a huge fraction of our energy needs are met by using oil, natural gas, gravity (hydroelectric dams), and nuclear reactors—all to make water flow so that it will do "work." We use these power sources to separate charges to create voltage to do work that we call electricity. But maybe all we need are commonly available hydrophilic surfaces such as gelatin proteins and water, with "flow" or "work" as the natural consequence. What could be more revolutionary than this?

Viktor Schauberger approached this subject from a different point of view. Schauberger came from a long line of foresters dating back to the thirteenth century, and he grew up living in and observing the rhythms and activities of the forest. He was especially interested in the waters that live in and flow through the forest. Many books, articles, and videos have covered his insights into water, his many inventions, and his work on energy generation and agriculture. And many practical applications of his discoveries are still in use today, especially in flow form technologies and agricultural tools. For many years, I have used copper tools in my garden and a vortex apparatus to structure my family's drinking water, both inspired by Schauberger.

In terms of understanding how blood flows in the human body, Schauberger made a few important observations that shed light on this process. The first is that for a stream or river to be healthy—for it to have clean, pure water that flows continuously and supports varied and abundant plant and animal life—it has to have two attributes. The first is that the flow pattern of the water in the stream or river must be in a vortex or spiral pattern. The second is that the temperature of the water, particularly at night, must be very close to or exactly at 4°C— the temperature that water is most likely to exist in the fourth, or structured, phase.[5]

The clue that both of these conditions are being met can be found by observing the habits of trout living in streams. When the water is healthy, Schauberger said, this results in a balance of the forces of gravity with the forces of levity.[6] Therefore, trout hanging out within the vortices upstream of the boulders in the stream could remain motionless indefinitely in the balance of these two forces. Suspended motionless in the stream, they allow the nutrients to come to them. The trout only move or exert themselves when it's time to spawn (when I first read Schauberger's account, I couldn't help but think this was eerily similar to a lot of men I know). The trout living this life of bliss were fat, tasty, and full of life-giving nutrition. Once, as Schauberger was patrolling the forest in the dead of night, he saw and described an amazing phenomenon: "In a suitably formed waterfall this energy flow can be distinguished as a channel of light within the streaming water, it is this energy that is used by the trout."[7]

When one lives almost entirely in nature that is unspoiled by human contact, one often develops strong powers of observation. What Schauberger saw is the force of levity that lives in water. This force of levity flows upward in vortices in the river. It is in these force "lines" that healthy trout live their effortless lives. Of course, these factors only exist when certain conditions are met. That is, the forest must be intact, there must be continuous tree covering shading the stream, there must be no dams anywhere on the stream, and the stream must be allowed to flow in its own path, not a path constructed by water "experts." When all these conditions are met, one can observe the forces of levity balancing the forces of gravity, and, if in the river itself, one can experience the blissful life of the trout.

When the forests are cut down and the streams are straightened and dredged, the forces of levity are lost, and the trout has to swim for its life to maintain its position in the stream. Too exhausted to swim by muscle power upstream, it ends up with a life of continuous and useless toil. This is not unlike the plight of industrial man, swimming upstream for his entire life, getting depleted, weaker, and sicker by the day.

The important point here is that this force of levity, which allows for the effortless flow of water, is dependent on certain conditions such as temperature and flow dynamics (spiral- or vortex-based flow patterns). When these conditions are met, life is easy and health is the natural outcome. This state is the natural state of structured water. It is also the natural state of the structured water that is the basis for the flow of blood in our circulatory system.

Combining Schauberger's understanding of the forces of levity with Pollack's work on the flow characteristics of structured water gives us insight into how fluids flow in living systems. Putting aside blood circulation for a moment, consider how and why sap flows up from the ground to the top of a 300-plus-foot redwood tree. Conventional science tells us that water cannot flow through a capillary tube more than 33 feet high before gravity prevents any further upward flow; this is known as the barometric limit. Yet there are many trees much taller than 33 feet, and sap flows to the top of them. Transpiration pull can account for some additional upward flow but, even in a best-case scenario, not more than about 45 feet.[8] So what can account for this paradox?

The answer is that the trees' xylem channels are highly hydrophilic tubes, which have a layer of negatively charged structured water lining the tube. At the center of the xylem channel is bulk water full of dissolved nutrients and positively charged protons that repel each other, pushing the bulk water upward. This upward flow will continue for as long as the tube is continuous.

This is the force of levity. It happens most powerfully, as Schauberger postulated, at 4°C and if the flow within the tubes is a spiraling or vortex motion, which it is within the xylem of the trees due to the gentle motions of the tree trunk. This explanation underscores just how intricate, exact, and profound the ways of nature truly are. There are four phases of water, but for biological life two are most important: The structured water phase creates the electrical charge that does the work, and the juxtaposed bulk phase simply flows.

Where is the energy input that drives this system? If you do the above tube experiment in a completely lead-encased box, there is no flow within the hydrophilic tube. But if you expose the beaker with the tube of water inside to ambient sunlight or the infrared frequencies coming from the palms of our hands or the electromagnetic field of the Earth, the flow resumes. There are many sources of natural energy that drive this flow, but the most powerful is sunlight. Sunlight is free, abundant, and available to all plants. Sunlight charges the hydrophilic tubes and creates the electrically charged structured water, causing the bulk water within the tube to flow indefinitely, as if life were just a big, blissful, abundant dance.

It is easier now to imagine how blood flows in our arteries and veins. Start at that precise place and moment where the blood in the vast network of capillaries has stopped, the gases and nutrients have been exchanged, and the waste products have been picked up. The blood needs to flow upward, coalescing into larger and larger vessels until the venous blood reaches its destination of the heart. The small venules are very narrow hydrophilic tubes; they are exposed to sunlight (if you have any doubt that light travels through us, go into a dark room and hold a flashlight against your palm), they pick up the Earth's electromagnetic field, and hopefully they experience the warmth and touch of another human being or animal. As a result, they, too, form a tubular layer of structured water on the inside of the venules. At the center of this layer of structured water is the positively charged bulk water with squeezed protons repelling each other. The blood begins to move upward. It goes faster and faster as the large "field" coalesces into a raging central river. There are, of course, contributions to this upward movement from the squeezing of the muscles of the legs and arms, but they are mostly helpful to maintain the spiral movement that supports the flow. There are also valves that keep the blood from succumbing to gravity if there are weak moments in the flow. But the main revelation here is that this system of hydrophilic tubes energized by the ambient sunlight, Earth energy, and the infrared wavelengths emanating from other living beings is really all that is needed in any biological system for the maintenance of abundant, robust, perpetual flow. The bulk water carries the waste and nutrients, and the structured layer creates the voltage or energy that runs the system. Like all living systems, we are powered by the Earth and sun.

This model allows us to see the real cause of varicose veins, congestive heart failure, and poor circulation. These ailments occur when the structured layer fails to form properly. It is as if someone cut down our forest, kept us from the sun and Earth, and gave us poor quality nutrients and water.

This model also offers crucial insight into what causes erosion of the blood vessels, or atherosclerosis. Erosion or inflammation of the blood vessels is the process underlying atherosclerosis, which is thought to be the cause of heart disease (see chapter 7). Pollack refers to the thick, viscous structured layer lining the vessel as the exclusion zone because it excludes toxins, solutes, and other substances. It's my opinion that this layer protects the vessel from inflammatory damage. When the structured, protective gel layer is not formed properly, the vessel walls (mostly on the arterial or high-pressure side) become damaged and inflamed. They protect themselves from the high pressure by forming plaque.

The publication of *De Motu Cordis* by William Harvey in 1628 was the death knell for the concept of a vital force that propelled the blood in the human body. The theory that the heart was the force driving the movement of the blood in the human body was the first and crucial step toward the development of the mechanistic medical model that we use to this day. Although I don't question that Harvey had valuable insights into the working of the circulatory system in humans and animals, perhaps the physicians of antiquity were not as incorrect as we have been led to believe. Perhaps the unique properties of water, recently rediscovered, reveal that water is the carrier of life, and that these fourth phase properties are the true "vital" forces that propel our circulation. If this is so, maybe it is time that the mechanistic view of the human being gives way to a more accurate description of how a human being actually functions. Perhaps a realistic view of circulation and what really propels the movement of our blood can provide a starting point for our long overdue reconnection with the healing forces that reside within nature.

CHAPTER THREE

The Misery Index

On the day I graduated from Duke with a BS in zoology, I felt both liberated from a school system I had grown to loathe and concerned that I had no skills and no clue what to do next. I headed to San Francisco, lived rent free with some friends from Detroit, and floated around the city, up and down the coast, and through the nearby parks and forests. Eventually I began looking for work, but was—fortunately— unable to find a job.

I say fortunately because I'd been reading Ivan Illich's book *The Right to Useful Unemployment* and was struck by what he wrote about society's Misery Index. In classical economics, the Misery Index is a real thing—at least in so far as anything in classical economics is a "real thing." An economic indicator developed by American economist Arthur Okun, the Misery Index has been in use since the Truman administration and is calculated, roughly, by adding the unemployment rate to the inflation rate. A higher number on the index indicates a higher rate of societal misery. According to the Misery Index, Americans were far less miserable under President Johnson (6.77), President Kennedy (7.14), and President Clinton (7.8), than we were under President Ford (16.00) and President Carter (16.26). The greatest increases in societal misery occurred under Presidents Nixon and Carter. And the greatest decreases in societal misery occurred under Presidents Reagan and Truman.[1]

Illich's perspective on the whole thing was different. If you want to calculate the Misery Index for a society, the most important rate to factor in is the *employment* rate. In traditional and indigenous cultures—rapidly declining in number, though they are—few people hold "jobs" and yet many people are quite happy. In industrialized countries and countries that are frantically trying to become industrialized, however, there are high levels of employment and also high rates of misery. We see this bearing out today. It's just that it is being measured in a different way. For example, the World Health Organization predicts that by 2020, depression will be the second leading cause of the global burden of disease.[2] And there is growing evidence that depression is a disease of modernity. A 2012 study found that, "The growing burden of chronic diseases, which arise from an evolutionary mismatch between past human environments and modern-day living, may be central to rising rates of depression. Declining social capital and greater inequality and loneliness are candidate mediators of a depressiogenic social milieu. Modern populations are increasingly overfed, malnourished, sedentary, sunlight-deficient, sleep-deprived, and socially isolated. These changes in lifestyle each contribute to poor physical health and affect the incidence and treatment of depression."[3]

The jobbed are miserable because they have to work for money at jobs they mostly despise. The un-jobbed are miserable because they are deemed useless for not having a job. And for the record, Illich wasn't idealizing poverty. He was describing "modern poverty" as a phenomenon that's been nurtured and groomed by global industrial capitalism.

When I was twenty years old, this made a great deal of sense to me. In fact, it still does.

This being the case, my employment options were subject to rather strict self-imposed limitations, so I decided to apply to the Peace Corps to see if I could experience, firsthand, two things that had always interested me: traditional cultures and Africa. I was accepted into an agriculture program based in Ghana and made my way home to Michigan to begin training.

As part of the required physical for Peace Corps service, however, my doctor thought he detected something odd going on with my heart. I was referred to a cardiologist who diagnosed me with an enlarged heart and Wolff-Parkinson-White syndrome, a rare condition in which an extra electrical pathway between the heart's upper chambers (atria) and lower chambers (ventricles) results in an abnormal heart rhythm (tachycardia). He refused to clear me medically.

Desperate for what felt like my best opportunity to get out of the country and do something meaningful, I scrambled for another opinion. I found a cardiologist who simplified the diagnosis to supraventricular tachycardia (SVT), an abnormal heart rhythm related to improper electrical activity in the heart. Instead of the normal "electrical system" in which the impulse starts in the sinoatrial node (SA node) of the left atrium and then travels through a "wire" of nerve cells to the left ventricle, I was born with a second "wire connection" from the SA node to the ventricle. The problem arises when the impulse travels down this accessory pathway because it goes at an unusual rate—in my case about 180–200 beats per minute. When I was young, the impulse usually traveled down the normal pathway and all was fine—except after the kind of exertion I experienced during high school basketball practices. Even in that case, I could manage it with a few minutes of rest. I hadn't been poorly conditioned; I had a funny conduction system in my heart.

More important than a diagnosis, though, was the fact that this doctor cleared me to go to Africa. But because of the time that had lapsed, I could no long accept the post in Ghana. I was assigned a post in Swaziland to teach gardening at an elementary school in the most rural part of the country.

———◆———

When I arrived at my post in Swaziland a few months later, there was only one other white man for fifty miles around. He was a Rhodesian escapee from the military who wound up on a biodynamic farm in South Africa before landing in Swaziland. This man, Chris, had a little garden of his own and helped me establish our version of the only biodynamic garden in Swaziland at the local school. A half acre with a four meter by four meter vegetable plot for each of the students, we conceived of it as an integrated system based on building healthy soil with compost rather than chemical inputs. In reality, some plots were well tended and some not so well, and the day before we intended to start harvesting the beans, tomatoes, carrots, and lettuce, someone came through and stole it all. Our enthusiasm waned after that, and the garden was never the same, although I'm glad we did it nevertheless.

Chris also loaded me up with books. In the evenings, I returned to my room in the village chief's mud and thatch-roofed hut and read these books by candlelight. There was nothing much else to do in the village after the sun went down, so I devoured everything Chris gave me, especially the books by and about Rudolf Steiner, including some on anthroposophical medicine. The type of doctor that Steiner and his students described was the most fascinating thing I'd ever encountered.

Rudolf Steiner envisioned the human being as a three-part organism made of the nervous system centered in the head; the rhythmical system centered in the heart and lungs; and the metabolic system centered in the abdomen. Steiner also argued that healthy societal organization should reflect this same three-fold principle based on: (1) human rights and equality such that no person's voice or autonomy shall be repressed or controlled by anyone else, with decisions made by consensus; (2) artistic, intellectual, and cultural freedom such that every individual can pursue his or her own path in life without interference from a state or governing body; and (3) cooperative economics driven by a sense of brotherhood and mutual care for others.

Steiner didn't originate this threefold way of envisioning a healthy body. In his work, we hear echoes of the French Revolution battle cry: liberty (in the creative realm), fraternity (in the economic realm), and equality (in rights and governance). And we hear echoes of the judicial, legislative, and executive branches of American government. In fact, some scholars argue that the US Constitution was influenced by the Iroquois, who reportedly organized themselves along similar principles, sustaining themselves for hundreds of years while continuously improving the habitat in which they lived.[4] Of course, our American ideals were not only never realized, but they were tainted from the beginning. You can't speak of equality in one breath and issue orders to slaves in the next any more than you can talk about the pursuit of happiness and self-realization during the day while conducting a campaign of genocide at night. But it's not that these principles are bad; it's just that the implementation was flawed—resulting in an ailing, fragmented, broken body.

Steiner's vision of the world, while "out there" at times, is consistent and makes sense. For example, Steiner argued that evolution as we conceive it is nonsense. He said that in the beginning everything was one, and over time, aspects were whittled off and became the zebras, daffodils, *Echinacea*, and so on. Eventually, after all of the other species were carved away, the human being was left in the center of creation—Michelangelo sculpting his David.

Medicine, according to Steiner, is a kind of reunification. The *Strophanthus* plant, for example, according to Steiner, was carved off at the same time as the human heart was forming. If you have an ailing heart, you need to be made whole—the etymological root of the word "heal"—so you need to find the part of the world, out there, that corresponds to that which is lacking in here, within your body. The metal antimony, or stibium, forms a long intricate molecular pattern, embodying "forces of cohesion" in nature. These forces of cohesion are lacking in a person with hemophilia or diarrhea, so one anthroposophical preparation for a person suffering in either of these ways would involve antimony to reunify and create wholeness.[5]

There in the mud hut, poring through the pages of Chris's books and as far from the influence of home and the United States as I could possibly be, it became clear to me that this was a coherent, plausible way to see the world, unlike anything I'd encountered in my life until that point. Anthroposophical medicine, I thought, at least tries to answer the real questions. I felt both revolted by the idea of becoming a doctor and also powerfully drawn to it. I suddenly knew that though my future was in medicine and in healing, it could not be on a conventional path.

Midway into my tour, I attended a gardening workshop on a farm near Manzini, Swaziland. The leader knew a lot about food, a subject I had been deeply interested in since my late teens when I started to eat only organic and mostly vegetarian food. After I peppered him with questions, he went inside his house, came out with a book and said, "Read this. It will answer all your questions."

The book was *Nutrition and Physical Degeneration*, by Weston A. Price. Originally published in 1939, the book is now considered a bible of modern nutrition.[6] It inaugurated the modern whole foods movement and spawned The Weston A. Price Foundation, of which I have been a board member since its inception in 1999. Weston Price on food and Rudolf Steiner on everything else were to be central pillars for the rest of my life.

———◆———

There were canoe trips in Africa, like those of my youth in northern Ontario: twice to the Okavango swamps in northern Botswana. But then it was home again with a clear sense of what was next—medical school to get in a position to pursue anthroposophical medicine, food as medicine, and whatever else my heart would lead me to.

CHAPTER FOUR

The Geometry of the Heart

I n chapter 2, I challenged the idea that the heart is a pump by looking at a different force within the body that circulates blood through the vessels. But if the heart is not a pump, what *is* it? If its purpose isn't to pump blood through the body, then what *is* the heart's purpose? What does it do? What happens to blood within the heart? What does the heart do with, or to, the blood? These are important questions about the heart's function. But we really can't begin to understand the heart's function without considering the heart's form.

What do we know about the structure of the heart? Well, the first thing is that the heart is not "heart-shaped"—as in Valentine's Day heart-shaped. I know this seems obvious, but I can still remember the day in anatomy class when I was slightly taken aback to discover that there was nothing about the heart in front of me that resembled a Valentine's Day heart. Of course, I'd seen beautiful images of organs in anatomy books, so I also half-expected to find a clearly outlined, well-defined organ in front of me. Instead, the heart in front of me looked like a lump of tissue. Not an organ, just tissue—a muscle, embedded in fat. Nonspecific, nondescript fat. I hid my disappointment, but a little part of me felt crushed. The heart was nothing special.

While in medical school, I learned that the heart is made out of a special kind of intermediate muscle (shared only by the uterus in the human body), that it has four valves each with its own set of "leaflets," and that each of the heart's four chambers—two upper atria and two lower ventricles—have a different thickness. We went on to examine the pressures and some aspects of the flow of blood entering and leaving the heart. But nothing was said about the actual shape of the heart. Or any other organ. This was simply not a matter of interest.

This lack of attention paid to the structure of the heart surprises me now because humans have a rich history of fascination with the human form and the geometry of the natural world. We see this in the depiction of people and various animals as a series of triangles and circles in ancient cave paintings. And we also see it in the writing of the ancient Greeks, especially that of Plato, who believed that the five Platonic solids—tetrahedron, cube, octahedron, dodecahedron, and icosahedron—were the basis of all natural phenomena, including of the human form. In fact, the architects and builders of antiquity were more or less obsessed with form. They were also amazingly precise. According to some sources, the precision of the base of the pyramids exceeds even that of our current capabilities.

One form that shows up again and again, both in nature and in human creations, is the spiral. In particular, there are many "golden" spirals in nature—a spiral whose growth factor is the golden ratio (1.618 expressed as a decimal, and represented as *phi*)—"golden" because the ratio is the same as the ratio of the sum to the larger of the two quantities. The Fibonacci series—the series of numbers you get when you add the previous two numbers together to obtain the next number in the series (1, 1, 2, 3, 5, 8, 13, 21, 34, 55 . . .)—approaches this golden ratio asymptotically.

The golden spiral shows up in the smallest of entities, such as DNA molecules, and in the most massive of entities, such as the Milky Way galaxy. Think, for example, of a nautilus shell or a fiddlehead. We see this golden spiral formation of leaves growing on branches, in the formation of rose petals, sunflower heads, snail shells, and on and on. The golden spiral can be seen in the Greek Parthenon, and the Fibonacci series can be heard in the first movement of Beethoven's fifth symphony.

When we turn to the human body, if we know how to look, we see number patterns, geometric forms, spirals, and Fibonacci numbers throughout our anatomy, as well. Consider the arrangement of our teeth. During the first part of our life, we have four sets of five baby teeth. Starting around age seven and ending around age twenty-one, we develop the full four sets of eight teeth. Perhaps it is not a coincidence that young children resonate most strongly with music in the five-note pentatonic scale until about the age of seven; in fact, most successful lullabies are written in the pentatonic scale. As adults, we leave the dreamy, pentatonic world and arrive at the octave, or eight-note scale.[1]

Or consider the relationship of the eight bones that reach from the shoulder to the tip of your fingers, or from your hip to your toes. The length of these bones is the same ratio as the intervals that lie between the notes on the western octave scale.[2] Are these coincidences? Or do they suggest an underlying strength or enhancement of function when structures are laid out according to geometric principles? Are there deeper creative principles at work here that are crucial to our understanding of how the body functions?

Understanding the form of something can offer crucial insight into its function. Take an egg, for example. Depending on the species, eggs vary somewhat in shape. Some are more conical and others are more spherical. Birds that nest on cliffs or in other precarious locations tend to lay more conical eggs because if they roll out of the nest, the eggs will roll in an arc rather than in a straight line (off the cliff!), whereas birds that make their homes in deep, well-protected nests tend to lay more spherical eggs. Tapered or not, an egg shape is one of the strongest forms in nature—resistant to breakage when subjected to pressure—so when something needs to protect its offspring, nature often puts those offspring inside of eggs.

It's important that we begin to rectify the kind of oversight that I encountered in medical school and gain a better understanding of the principles nature uses to create form, and what form can then teach us about function. This is complicated, to be sure, and it's easy to indulge in almost delusional revelations about the significance of things that turn out to be nothing at all. Maybe this is part of why the discussion is avoided altogether in medical school: it's seen as too "woo-woo." But it's a shame that we then completely avoid this rich, crucial, and potentially lifesaving subject for fear that the medical profession would look less serious or would appear too "out there," and that for the sake of our careers, we avoid all mention (or even thought!) of deeper meaning or connections. The unfortunate consequence is that we have only a superficial understanding of nature, the body, and the magic of seeing a big picture relationship between the two.

My investigation into the shape of the heart didn't really begin until I encountered the brilliant work of a contemporary San Francisco–based Waldorf teacher, sculptor, geometrician, and philosopher named Frank Chester. Chester's interest is in forms found in nature and how they can be transformed into works of art. In 2000, following a class he took at Rudolf Steiner College, Chester became particularly interested in the Platonic solids—the three-dimensional geometric forms that Plato thought were the basis of all natural phenomena.

These five Platonic solids are unique and fascinating because they are the only "regular" convex polyhedrons. A "regular" polygon, for anyone who might legitimately need a high school geometry refresher, is a two-dimensional figure that is equiangular (that is, all its angles are equal) and equilateral (that is, all its sides are equal). So a regular polyhedron, or Platonic solid, is a three-dimensional form that is equiangular and equilateral. A cube, for example, is a common Platonic solid, or regular, convex polyhedron.

Through his knowledge of anthroposophy, Chester knew that, according to some people, Steiner had described the heart as a seven-sided form that sits in an imaginary box in the chest. Chester became intrigued with this idea and wondered if anyone

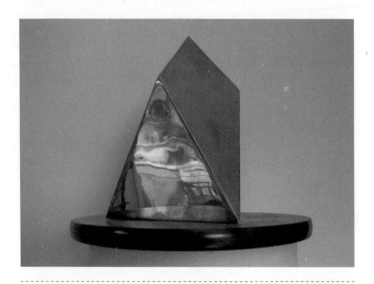

Frank Chester's chestahedron is a seven-sided form made of four equilateral triangles and three kite-shaped quadrilaterals. The chestahedron has equivalent surface areas as—twelve edges, three different symmetries—and may offer insight into the form and function of the human heart. Reproduced with permission from Frank Chester, New Form Technology, http://www.frankchester.com/.

had ever tried to model such a thing. He set out to sculpt this form. After many failed attempts, Frank succeeded in sculpting a chestahedron: a seven-sided form of four equilateral triangles and three kite-shaped quadrilaterals with equivalent surface areas, twelve edges, and three different symmetries. This seemingly humble achievement offers some dramatic insights into the form and function of the human heart.

Frank's next step, as Steiner might have suggested, was to put this seven-sided form into a box—that is, the tightest cube it could fit into. In other words, imagine taking this form, facing the point down and just fitting it into a "regular" box. The apex, or point, does not fall in the center of the cube, but rather slightly off-center. Specifically, the chestahedron sits at an angle of 36 degrees off of center.[3] Amazingly, this is the same angle at which the heart sits within the chest: 36 degrees off center to the left of the midline.[4]

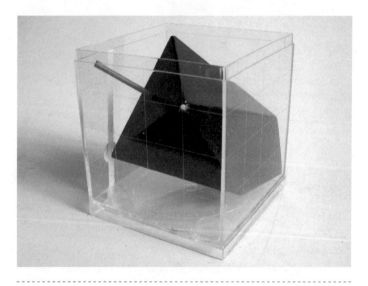

When placed in a box, the chestahedron sits at an angle of 36 degrees off center. This is the same angle at which the heart sits within the chest. Image courtesy of Frank Chester.

Chester was intrigued about what other insights into the human heart this seven-sided form might reveal. He discovered that if you slightly round off the edges of a chestahedron of proportional size, it will fit precisely into the cavity of the left ventricle, the largest chamber of our four-chambered heart. Indeed, it is the left ventricle that gives us the 36-degree angle of the heart in the chest. So now we have the inner form of the left ventricle, sitting at the same angle as the chestahedron does in a cube-shaped box.

Not stopping there, Frank then made a wire model of the chestahedron, put it into a vat of water, and spun it. The spinning chestahedron formed a vortex—a region where the flow forms around an axis line—in the water. Once the vortex formed, an area appeared in the water, a kind of negative space that appeared attached to the side of the chestahedron. (You can really appreciate this only by seeing the video of this on Frank's website.[5])

Perplexed at first, and doing something only a master sculptor could do or probably even think of doing, Frank sculpted the form of the whirling chestahedron with its attached "appendix." He found that this appendix creates its own vortex when spun in water, but more horizontally, rather than the more vertically shaped vortex created by the chestahedron itself. This more horizontal vortex itself closely resembles the shape and attachment of the right ventricle to the left ventricle of a human heart. Chester then took a cross section of the spinning chestahedron, including its attachment near the thickest area and, again amazingly, this reproduced a similar cross section of both the right and left ventricle of the heart. The wall thicknesses are the same, the size of the cavities is the same, and the angles of attachment of the ventricles and the forms are nearly identical.

I can only imagine the sense of awe and wonder Frank Chester must have felt when he first realized what he had discovered and created. Could it be that the human heart is a seven-sided form within a cube-shaped box in the chest, just as Steiner predicted?

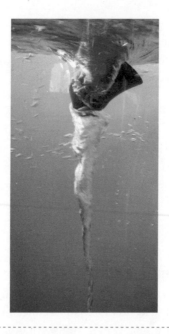

Spinning the chestahedron will form a vortex. Once the vortex forms, an area appears in the water, a kind of negative space that appears attached to the side of the chestahedron. This "appendix" creates its own vortex when spun in water but more horizontal than the vertically shaped vortex created by the chestahedron itself. This more horizontal vortex resembles the shape and attachment of the right ventricle to the left ventricle of a human heart. Image courtesy of Frank Chester.

But these aren't the only insights we can gain from studying the chestahedron in relation to the heart. Back in anatomy class, I learned that the heart is a muscle and that the thickness of the muscle varies in different parts of the heart. But I never learned how many layers of muscle the heart has. Nor did we investigate why the apex—the bottom of the heart where the point of the upside-down chestahedron meets the bottom of the cube—is so thin. The apex is *one* muscle layer thick. This is the point in the heart that sits directly opposite the outlet of the left ventricle, the aortic valve. In the pump model of the heart, this should be the area of most stress or tension. How is it possible that, just at this area of maximum stress, it is so thin?

Still on his investigative path, Frank Chester encountered the anatomical work of Dr. James Bell Pettigrew, a nineteenth-century Scottish naturalist, who conducted detailed dissections of the layers of muscles of the heart. Dr. Pettigrew found that at various points in the heart, the number of layers of muscle varies from a minimum of one (at the apex) to seven.[6] Working with the geometric knowledge he'd gained, Chester began wrapping his spinning chestahedron in layers of paper at the angles outlined by the cones of water created by the spinning chestahedron in water. (These are different from the vortex created by the spinning wire form.) The only way Chester could properly wrap the form—while still maintaining the outline of the spinning form—also reproduced the thickness of the muscle layers at the various points of the heart: seven layers at the thickest and one layer at the apex.[7]

We can now return to the opening question of this chapter: What does the heart do, and what happens to the blood inside the heart? We know so far that due to the recently observed unique properties of water, in particular its ability to exist in a fourth phase, the blood in the venous system flows upward toward the heart, essentially under its own power. (Again, there is some contribution from the valves and muscle contraction.) This mainly vertical flow arrives at the right atrium, the small chamber above the right ventricle.

When Rudolf Steiner was pressed to suggest a more appropriate mechanical image for the heart than a pump, Steiner replied that the closest "machine" to the heart is a hydraulic ram. A hydraulic ram is a device that is primarily placed in flowing water; it holds the water in a holding tank behind its gating mechanism. When the pressure and volume build up on the incoming side of the gate, a vacuum, or negative pressure, is created on the far side of the gate. At a certain pressure differential across the gate, the gate will open, and the fluid can be propelled up the hill.

Something similar happens in the heart. The venous blood flows into the right atrium, the pressure in the right atrium builds up, then the gate (the tricuspid valve) opens, and the blood enters the right ventricle. But this isn't all that happens. As the chestahedron model shows, fluid arriving into the right ventricle converts into a vortex before emerging out of the next gate (the pulmonary valve). This is the crucial point. There are two processes happening simultaneously. The first is the increase in momentum due to the hydraulic ram/gating mechanism described above. But along with the increase in momentum, the form of the blood changes from a laminar flow to a vortex. Furthermore, the activity of the right side of the heart converts the vertically oriented laminar flow of the venous blood to a vortex, a horizontal flow, as the blood goes from the right ventricle to the horizontally positioned lungs.

The blood then travels through the lungs, again moving into the capillaries as a result of water's—or, in this case, blood's—fourth phase tendency to flow within hydrophilic tubes. I have never heard any other remotely possible explanations of how or why blood can move through the high-resistance environment of the lung capillaries. Remember that you have highly viscous blood with blood cells suspended in plasma and whose diameter is almost as large as the capillaries moving effortlessly through an extensive network of lung capillaries. Attributing this to the low pump pressure of the right ventricle would be like taking a mile-long hose, putting water and beads inside the hose where the beads are about the same size as the internal dimensions of the hose, giving a little push, and expecting the water and beads to travel a half mile—and then return the half mile back to the pump.

After the blood flows into the capillaries, it then continues its now horizontal flow back to the left atrium of the heart, which serves as a temporary holding area to store the energy of the flowing blood behind the mitral valve. The pressure builds up in the left atrium, the gate opens, and the blood flows into the left ventricle. Then—think now of the spinning chestahedron in water—the left ventricle converts this laminar flow into a vertically oriented vortex. This vortex flow, combined with the pressure buildup, opens the aortic valve, and the blood is released through the arteries to the rest of the body.

Further evidence that the best model for the heart is a hydraulic ram and not a pump is the behavior of the aortic arch during contraction, known as systole. If the heart were a pump, you would expect that as the heart pumps blood through the aortic arch, the flexible arch would straighten with each forceful push. On the contrary, however, during this contraction, the aortic arch bends inward, forming a more acute angle. This can be seen on a routine angiogram.

Imagine putting a flexible garden hose on your outside spigot. Attach the hose to the spigot and shape the hose into an arch soon after it emerges from the spigot. Then quickly turn the spigot on to full flow, causing a forceful stream of water to emerge. What would you expect the flexible arch of the hose to do? The arch would straighten under the increased force, but this is the opposite of what happens in our aortic arch. Each time we expect the force to increase in systole, the arch bends in. This bending in during systole can only be explained by a *negative* pressure, and this negative pressure is akin to the suction created by a hydraulic ram. In other words, this anomalous behavior of the aortic arch demonstrates that rather than pushing blood under force, the heart is creating negative pressure, or suction. The action of the heart on the blood is not one of creating force, but instead of using suction to increase the momentum of the blood.

CHAPTER FIVE

Defining the Questions

B y 1983, I was in my third year of medical school, had already completed my two years in the Peace Corps in Swaziland, and was the new father of a one-year-old girl. I was also already full of enthusiasm for two ideas that would inform my work for decades to come: food as medicine and anthroposophy, the spiritual-science philosophy of Rudolf Steiner. That year, I had the opportunity to attend my first anthroposophical conference—an annual doctor's training week held at an anthroposophical community in Wilton, New Hampshire.

At the time, my only exposure to anthroposophy had been through books, but I was nevertheless certain that I was onto some major insights that would enable me to treat and cure any disease that might come my way once I became a full-fledged physician. Overall, I was bursting with life.

During the first evening of the conference, I attended a lecture by Francis Edmunds, a Russian-born English teacher who was a leader in the Waldorf School movement. I had never heard a lecture like his before. It left me in awe that someone could speak with such vigor, such clarity, and such force even though he was in his eighties at the time. It also left me with a profound sense of sadness. I had been through eighteen years of schooling and had heard thousands of lectures, but this was the first time I listened to a lecture that rang true, that had this kind of power, and that spoke directly to my heart.

Now, more than thirty years later, I can barely remember what Edmunds even talked about that night, but I do remember how impressed I was by the clarity with which he spoke about complex issues. Typically, now as then, when I hear someone, often a scientist, give a lecture, it's one study after another, statistics on what a study suggests, and how a given study adds to the body of knowledge. In its place, that's well and good. But it's one thing to hear about research suggesting that early play may improve young childhood development; it's another to listen to an eighty-year-old man with a crystal clear voice tell you that young children "grow" into the world. Edmunds didn't refer to anyone else's work or research. He simply offered his own insights, developed from a lifetime of work, observation, and contemplation. He needed no external validation—the listener could accept it or not. As I listened, I felt as though his words were coming from a different place—from, if I may be permitted some hyperbole, the land of knowing. It was so refreshing and so different that I've never forgotten the experience of sitting in the audience and listening to him.

That night, I made a decision—although I think it was largely subconscious—that I wanted to someday be able to speak from this place of knowing. I had a sense that learning anthroposophy would provide me with the path, but I also had a sense that I needed to deeply question everything I encountered and that to reach the land of knowing from which Francis Edmunds seemed to speak would not be a straight shot or an easy journey. I also sensed that it was the only journey worth taking.

The conference in Wilton was my first stop on a three-month journey with my wife and daughter so that I could learn anthroposophical medicine from three of the country's best practitioners, who had agreed to take me on as an apprentice. I was determined to prove to them that I was knowledgeable about medicine in general and anthroposophical medicine and natural medicine in particular. Then, as now, I hated feeling unprepared or feeling like someone else knew more than I did about a subject I was interested in. I can acknowledge this as a weakness and insecurity, but it's also been an asset to me in my life and was especially so when I was a young man. It drove me to understand and master things in a way that served me well.

The doctors had different styles. Richard Fried in Kimberton, Pennsylvania, ran a more or less conventional family practice with a strong anthroposophical bent. Phillip Incao in Copake, New York, was a real radical who focused a lot on diet and wanted no part of conventional medicine. We were provided housing in a Steiner-inspired village for developmentally disabled adults, most of whom had autism spectrum disorder. We ate meals with the family in whose home we were staying. The final apprenticeship was back in New Hampshire with Bertram Von Zabern, more of a psychiatrist and a philosopher.

All three liked having me around because I understood the theory and was already pretty well studied in how to see the world as an anthroposophist, so we could see a patient and then have a discussion about where the patient's real problem or imbalance lay and how to heal (read: reunify) him or her. It was all really fun, and it was before I started anthroposophical medicine myself and caught on that using conventional anthroposophical remedies didn't help me resolve my patients' issues as much as I had hoped or expected.

Throughout the rest of medical school and my residency, I mostly adopted an attitude of keeping very much to myself and preparing for whatever exams or tests were needed to keep me moving through the system. No one had any particular complaints about me, but I was often told I was hard to teach. From my perspective, I was there to learn the system, not to engage in debate about whether the system was right.

In the meantime, I attended week-long anthroposophical medical training sessions each year, where two important things happened for me. For the first time, I met a group of peers who were interested in the same subjects as I was—mostly medicine, food, and life in the deepest sense. The second, and maybe more important, thing is that I met someone whom I could accept as a teacher. The main person who came from Europe to start anthroposophical medicine in the United States was Otto Wolff, a German MD and PhD who, as far as I could tell, knew everything. He looked like Beethoven (as far as the descriptions of Beethoven are accurate) and he knew every star, every constellation, every plant, twelve languages, every mineral, every medicine—conventional, homeopathic, herbal, or anthroposophical—and spent his free time skydiving and exploring. He had been on a canoe trip to the Okavango swamps in Africa with the same guide on the same route as I had been on a few years earlier.

It was from Otto, who was not shy about questioning us and being impatient with us, that I learned about a different way of seeing and thinking about the world. Learning anthroposophy was like learning a new language, the language of artistic thinking. It is the thinking that asks why the blood moves the way it does, what happens in the heart, and how this is connected with the smallest particles or the furthest cosmic bodies. Always the words of Otto ring in my awareness, "Substance does nothing." For, to Otto, the universe and everything in it was a flowing, dynamic field of forces that he attempted to understand and describe in great detail.

It is the difference between studying how the forces of the cosmos shape the heart versus studying that the heart is made of specialized muscle cells called myocytes and that they contain actin tubules. Experiencing this way of thinking and, as Otto also said, to be an anthroposophical doctor, you have to know everything. You have to know sophisticated biochemistry, the names and stories of the constellations, the history of music (Otto was a highly proficient classical violinist), how to skydive, and the entire pharmacopeia (hundreds of pages) of anthroposophical medicines.

Otto inspired me to take up the recorder and painting, memorize the anthroposophical and homeopathic pharmacopeia, sing in a choir, and learn the metals, the constellations, plants, gardening, and the movement of water. While I never got much good at biochemistry and never tried to skydive, my eyes were opened on what a full human being should at least try to know and experience. This phase of my life was spent gathering questions: What moves the blood? Why do cells lose connection to each other and the larger whole and become "selfish"? At the time, I intently explored the nature of these forces Otto spoke of, wondering if they were real and, if so, how they worked.

As soon as I completed medical training, our family returned to New Hampshire, where I launched a practice in Peterborough based on anthroposophical medicine and healing through traditional foods. This combination, I thought, was enough to cure anything that afflicted my patients. One of the motivations behind our decision to return to New Hampshire was that I remained close with the farmers at the Waldorf community in Wilton, who were busy developing the first community-supported agriculture (CSA) in the country. I wanted to be a part of this personally and close to it so that my patients would have access to the best possible food. The farm and Waldorf School were also developing a gift economy, and eventually my medical practice would be largely supported in this way.

During this time, I saw myself as an evangelist for truth, on a journey in pursuit of the same passion and conviction I'd witnessed in Francis Edmunds. I developed dietary guidelines for patients and experimented with variations on it by tweaking the amounts of macronutrients—proteins, fats, and carbohydrates, for example. I tried new medicines, new movement and exercise strategies, and new ways of thinking about disease in general and the heart in particular. There were experiments with the ketogenic diet, water fasts, qi gong for movement, curative eurythmy, IV vitamin C, DMSO, canivora for cancer, oxygen therapies, and natural medicines of every stripe.

Although it was a time of learning and great experimentation—maybe *because* it was a time of learning and great experimentation—many explanations I consistently relied on began to feel hollow over time. Worse, most of my treatments failed to help my patients transform their lives. I began to search for ways to ground the insights I'd gained from anthroposophy into something more solid. Those insights, the footprints of which can be found throughout this book, have proven invaluable in my quest to understand the heart, but I realize now that I'd been expecting a unifying answer, enlightenment, a silver platter—once I gained mastery over the subject. And that expectation, I came to realize, was way too arrogant, simplistic, childish. The hard work of discovering what was real, what actually worked for my patients, and how insights from anthroposophy and elsewhere interfaced with conventional science and medicine had only just begun.

CHAPTER SIX

What Doesn't Cause Heart Attacks

I n writing this book, I wanted to start out by examining the physiology and anatomy of normal circulation and a healthy heart, as I've done in chapters 2 and 4, respectively. This is because I think mainstream medicine gets so much wrong—including a focus on "fixing" what is abnormal, diseased, and dysfunctional rather than really understanding how things should work and proceeding from there.

For example, if we want to understand the nature and spectrum of infectious disease, it would be wise for us to thoroughly examine and understand the role of microbial life in nature and in the human body. If we did so, we would know that microbes are not only a necessary part of every ecosystem but that humans can't survive without the seven or eight pounds of microbes that make their home in our intestines. We would understand that microbes are partly scavengers of dead matter (especially fungi), partly agents of digestion (mainly bacteria), and finally agents of modifying genetic materials (viruses). But rather than studying the intricacies of the interactions between microbes and other forms of life, or even how microbes contribute to and modify entire ecosystems, we start medical school by learning that the strep bacteria causes sore throats, its life cycle is such and such, and we kill it with penicillin. Next.

The culture around this paradigm is changing—albeit not quickly enough—but in medical training, there is still too much of a focus on wiping out the disease and not enough focus on understanding microbial communities and our coevolution with microbial ancestors, in the same way there isn't enough emphasis on studying the form and structure of our anatomy. But even though I favor a whole-systems, health-based approach to medicine rather than a reductionist, disease-centric approach, there's still no escaping the fact that a lot of people—and a lot of communities and ecosystems, too—are sick and in distress. And worldwide, the leading cause of death is heart disease.[1]

What does it mean for a heart to be diseased? Even if you completely discard metaphysical explanations (which I don't, and I will explore them in greater detail in chapters 10 and 11) and set aside the many diseases of the heart that don't fall under the umbrella of cardiovascular disease, the answer is still somewhat of a semantic challenge. That's because when doctors say "heart disease," they're often referring to events or conditions that happen in the coronary arteries (the arteries that supply the heart), such as coronary artery disease, which can block blood flow to the heart and lead to a heart attack. Or so the conventional wisdom says. The spectrum of heart disease that includes angina, unstable angina, and myocardial infarction (heart attack)—typically referred to as *coronary artery disease*—is actually much better understood from the perspective of events happening in the myocardium (heart), not events happening in the coronary arteries.[2]

This perspective is crucial because the coronary artery theory of heart disease has cost the nation billions of dollars in surgical costs (mostly unnecessary, I argue) and billions in medications that cause as much harm as good, and has led many people to adopt a low-fat diet, which worsens the problem. According to the Centers for Disease Control and Prevention, about 735,000 Americans suffer heart attacks each year. And nearly 610,000 Americans die each year from heart disease, accounting for one in every four deaths.[3] The CDC Foundation estimates that heart disease and strokes cost Americans nearly $1 billion per day in medical costs and lost productivity, and projects that, by 2030, annual direct medical costs will exceed $818 billion and lost productivity could exceed $275 billion.[4]

By understanding the real pathophysiological events behind heart attacks, we can adopt a heart-healthy diet (by which I mean a Weston A. Price–type diet, not a low-fat diet), the use of safe and inexpensive medicine (such as g-strophanthin), and other nontoxic and effective therapies. Most importantly, understanding the events in the heart that precede a heart attack will force us to look at how heart disease is a manifestation of the true cost of modern life to human health. To overcome the epidemic of heart disease, we will need a new medical paradigm, a new economic system, and a new ecological consciousness—in short, a new way of life. The coronary artery theory misses this larger picture, just as it misinterprets the actual pathological events.

Because conventional medicine gets so much wrong about the heart, I want to start with the definition of a heart attack. In this definition, I don't take much issue with conventional medicine. A heart attack, or myocardial infarction, is an event that leads to the death of myocardial cells (heart cells). The death of these myocardial cells leads then to necrosis of the tissue. The myocardial infarction is diagnosed by an elevation of cardiac enzymes that normally reside inside the cells of your heart. When these cells die, they lyse (break), releasing their contents, including the enzymes, into the blood.

Beyond this definition of a heart attack, the semantics of heart disease are challenging because the language is skewed toward blood flow. And you can't accurately refer to *heart disease* because that doesn't distinguish between heart attacks, rhythm problems, congestive heart failure, and so on. Rather than *heart disease*, many people use *coronary heart disease*, but this suggests that heart disease is caused by the coronary arteries. I often refer to the spectrum of illnesses as *angina, unstable angina*, and *myocardial infarction*. Although this is cumbersome wording, it's typically what I'm referring to when I discuss the type of disease that includes heart attacks.

Until recently, it was thought that most heart attacks were caused by progressive blockage created by plaque buildup in the major arteries leading to the heart. The plaque was thought to be cholesterol buildup in the arterial lumen (inside of the vessel), which eventually cut off blood supply to a certain area of the heart, resulting in oxygen deficiency in that area, causing first pain (angina), then progressing to myocardial infarction (heart attack). The simple solution was to clear the stenosis (blockage) with either an angioplasty or a stent, or, if that was not possible, to bypass the area with coronary bypass grafting. Simple problem, simple solution.

However, problems with this theory began to emerge. A major report on the efficacy of bypasses, stents, and angioplasty that was issued by the Mayo Clinic in 2003[5] concluded that:

1. Bypass surgery relieves symptoms (chest pain).
2. Bypass surgery does not prevent future heart attacks.
3. Only high-risk patients, those whose life is in acute danger, benefit from bypass surgery (i.e., have improved chances of survival).

In other words, the gold standard for treating arterial blockages—surgery—has, at best, only minimal benefits. This is because large, stable blockages—those that block more than 90 percent of the vessel—are in almost 100 percent of the cases completely compensated for by collateral blood vessels.[6] In fact, the idea that the heart gets its blood only from the four major vessels is not correct. Starting soon after birth, the normal heart develops an extensive network of small blood vessels called collateral vessels, which compensate for the interruption of flow in any one (or more) of the major vessels. This compensation by collateral vessels can be seen clearly in a video ("Heart Catheter Film") produced by Dr. Knut Sroka for his website www.heart attacknew.com.

As Sroka correctly points out in his video, coronary angiogram—which fails to show the collateral circulation and creates spasms in the coronary arteries through the injection of heavy dye under high pressure—is a notoriously inaccurate tool for assessing the amount of stenosis in the vessels and the amount of blood flow in the heart. Most bypasses, stents, and angioplasties are performed on minimally symptomatic patients who show a greater than 90 percent blockage in one or more coronary arteries. These arteries are almost always fully collateralized; the surgery does not restore blood flow because the body had already done its own bypass. Ask yourself: If it were true that an artery that was more than 90 percent blocked had no collateral circulation, how is that person still alive? Does it make sense that a person would have a heart attack when the stenosis goes from 93 percent to 98 percent? Yet this is what most of the procedures are meant to accomplish—to unblock the stenosis—which, as Sroka's video shows, actually has no effect on the amount of blood flow. It is no wonder that in study after study, these procedures fail to provide any significant benefit to patients.

For example, at a conference I attended and presented at in Northern California, a cardiologist reported about a trial he helped conduct in rural Alabama during his residency. In this trial, angiograms—injections of dye into the coronary arteries to detect blockages—were done on men presenting with chest pains. For the ones who had a single artery blocked, no treatment was prescribed, and the researchers predicted in their notes which part of the heart would have a subsequent heart attack if one occurred. Of course, all of the researchers predicted that the heart attack would take place in the part of the heart supplied by the blocked coronary artery. Many of the men did eventually have heart attacks, but to the researchers' surprise, fewer than 10 percent had a heart attack in the area of the heart supplied by the original blocked artery.

For these reasons, the stable-plaque model is being abandoned by conventional cardiology in favor of a different model for the etiology of MIs, which, as it turns out, is almost equally invalid.

So, most of us can pretty much now agree that the long-standing focal point of cardiology—the stable, progressing, calcified plaque, the thing we bypassed and stented for years, the thing we do CT scans of your arteries for, the thing we told you is from cholesterol buildup in your arteries, the thing low-fat, high-carbohydrate, largely vegetarian diets such as the Ornish Program focused on—is actually not that important in the etiology of heart attacks.

But conventional medical thinking is still focused on the arteries. Enter the unstable, or friable, plaque. This insidious fellow doesn't actually create a large blockage; rather, it's a soft, "foamy" plaque that under certain situations (we don't know which situations) rapidly evolves and abruptly closes off the involved artery, creating a downstream oxygen deficit, followed by angina, then ischemia (a restriction of the blood supply). These soft plaques are thought to be a combination of inflammatory "buildup" and LDL, the two things we target with statin drugs. Therefore, the thinking goes, because this type of plaque can build up in anyone's arteries, at any time, everyone should be on statin drugs to prevent heart attacks. (Some people even advocate putting therapeutic doses of statins in municipal water supplies.[7]) Angiogram studies are used to show the evolution of these unstable plaques as proof that they are the true cause of most heart attacks.

When a person suffers a heart attack, there is often the formation of a blood clot within a vessel of the heart (acute thrombosis), but it is a *consequence*, not the cause, of the attack. How often does this actually happen? Well, first off, it's critical to look to pathology studies, which are the only accurate way to determine what actually happened, as opposed to angiograms, which are misleading and create many artifacts. Anytime you put heavy metal dye under high pressure into an artery (which is what an angiogram is), the artery reacts with a spasm. So imagine you have an artery, of which 50 percent of the cross section of the interior is blocked with plague. Then you push heavy dye into the artery, which causes the muscle wall of the artery to go into spasm; suddenly the interior dimension is narrower, but the amount of plaque doesn't change, so it looks as though the plaque is blocking 70 percent or more of the artery. This is an "artifact" due to the spasm-inducing tendency of the test itself, which then leads to overattribution of the percentage of stenosis, or blockage.

The first major pathology study of people who died of heart attacks was conducted in the 1970s. It concluded that stenosis sufficient to cause the heart attack was found in only 20 percent of cases.[8] And in the largest such study ever done, examining the autopsies of patients who died of heart attacks—the results of which were published in 2004—Giorgio Baroldi and Malcolm D. Silver found sufficient stenosis to cause the heart attack in 41 percent of cases.[9] They also found that the larger the area of necrosis, the more often a stenosis was present, and the longer the time between heart attack and death, the higher the percentage of stenosis—two findings that some subsequent researchers have used to artificially inflate the stenosis rates by focusing only on the cases of very significant heart attacks or those in which the patients lived a relatively long time after the event.

There's another reason to doubt the coronary artery etiology paradigm of heart attacks. In this paradigm, blocked arteries cause ischemia by cutting off the blood supply, thereby cutting off the supply of oxygen to the tissues. But when careful measurements assessing the oxygen (pO2) of the myocardial cells during a heart attack are taken, they show no oxygen deficit in an evolving heart attack.[10] The oxygen levels do not change at all throughout the entire event. (I will return to this concept in chapter 7 when I describe what *does* change in every evolving heart attack ever studied.) If a coronary artery blockage is the mechanism by which the oxygen supply is cut off to the myocardial cells, but, in fact, the oxygen supply to the heart doesn't change, then what exactly does happen to result in tissue necrosis in the heart?

Thrombosis associated with heart attacks is a real phenomenon, but in no pathological study has it been found in more than 50 percent of deaths, which begs the question: Why did the other 50 percent have a heart attack? Furthermore, it's clear from pathology studies that thrombosis of significant degrees often evolves *after* the attack occurs, leading again to the question of what caused the heart attack in the first place. The fact that thrombosis correlates with heart attacks does explain why emergency procedures can be helpful immediately following a heart attack to restore blood flow in those patients who do not have adequate collateral circulation to that part of their heart. (Remember, the only patients who benefit from bypass and stents are the most critical, acute patients.) But if the coronary artery etiology paradigm of heart attacks is so fraught with inconsistencies and if it provides such an imperfect and unpersuasive explanation for the cause of heart attacks, the question remains: What *does* cause heart attacks?

CHAPTER SEVEN

What Does Cause Heart Attacks

A ny accurate theory of the cause of myocardial infarction must account for the risk factors most associated with heart disease and heart attacks. These are being male, having diabetes, smoking cigarettes, and experiencing chronic psychological/emotional stress. Significantly, none of these risk factors is directly linked to pathology of the coronary arteries. Diabetes and cigarette use cause disease in the capillaries, not the large vessels, and stress has no direct effect on coronary arteries that we know of. Additionally, during the past five decades, the four main medicines of modern cardiology (beta-blockers, nitrates, aspirin, and statin drugs) all have some benefits for heart patients—albeit, all with serious drawbacks as well. This also needs to be accounted for in any comprehensive theory of the cause of heart attacks.

The real revolution in the prevention and treatment of heart disease has to do with the autonomic nervous system. First, let's review some brief (and admittedly oversimplified) background. We have two distinct nervous systems. The central nervous system controls conscious functions such as that of muscles and nerves. The autonomic (or unconscious) nervous system controls the function of our internal organs.

The autonomic nervous system is divided into two branches, which in health are always in a balanced, but ready, state. The sympathetic, or fight-or-flight, system is centered in our adrenal medulla and uses the chemical adrenaline to tell our bodies that danger is afoot. It does so by activating a series of biochemical responses, the center of which are the glycolytic pathways that accelerate the breakdown of glucose to be used as quick energy so that we can make our escape.

In contrast, the parasympathetic branch is centered in the adrenal cortex and uses the neurotransmitters acetylcholine, nitric oxide, and cyclic guanosine monophosphate as its chemical mediators. It is the rest-and-digest arm of the autonomic nervous system. The particular nerve of the parasympathetic chain that innervates the heart is called the vagus nerve. It slows and relaxes the heart, whereas the sympathetic branch accelerates and constricts the heart. It is the imbalance of these two branches that is responsible for most heart disease.

Using heart-rate variability monitoring, which offers a real-time, accurate depiction of these two branches of the autonomic nervous system, four studies have shown that patients with ischemic heart disease have, on average, a reduction of parasympathetic activity of more than a third.[1] Typically, the worse the myocardial infarction, the lower the parasympathetic activity.[2]

Furthermore, about 80 percent of ischemic events are preceded by chronic reductions in parasympathetic activity, which can be brought on by smoking, emotional stress, inactivity, poor diet, hypertension, or—often—a combination of these, followed by a significant, often drastic increase in sympathetic activity such as an acute traumatic event or physical exertion.[3] People who have normal parasympathetic activity and then experience an abrupt increase in sympathetic activity (physical activity or, often, an emotional shock) don't suffer from heart infarction. In other words, without a preceding decrease in parasympathetic activity, activation of the sympathetic nervous system does not lead to myocardial infarction.[4] Human beings are meant to experience, and are fully capable of experiencing, times of excess sympathetic activity; that is normal life. What's dangerous to our health is the ongoing, persistent decrease in our parasympathetic, or life-restoring, activity.

It has been shown that women have stronger vagal activity than men, probably accounting for the sex difference in the incidence of myocardial infarction.[5] Hypertension, smoking, diabetes, and physical and emotional stress all cause a decrease in vagal activity.[6] In other words, all the significant risk factors have been shown to downregulate the activity of the regenerative nervous system in our heart.

On the other hand, the main drugs used in cardiology—nitrates—stimulate nitrous oxide production, which upregulates the parasympathetic nervous system. Aspirin and statin drugs also stimulate the production of nitric oxide and acetylcholine, two of the principal mediators of the parasympathetic nervous system—until they cause a rebound decrease in these substances, which then further reduces parasympathetic activity. Finally, beta-blockers (used to manage cardiac arrhythmias and prevent second heart attacks) are called beta-blockers because they block the activity of the sympathetic nervous system. In other words, these interventions all help balance the autonomic nervous system. As with the risk factors, their effect on plaque and stenosis development is of minor relevance.

So, what is the sequence of events that leads to a heart attack?

In the vast majority of cases, the pathology proceeds because of decreased tonic activity of the parasympathetic nervous system. Then there is an increase in sympathetic nervous system activity, usually due to a physical or emotional stressor. This increases adrenaline production, which directs the myocardial cells to break down glucose using aerobic glycolysis. (Remember, there has been no change in blood flow as measured by the oxygen in the cells.) This redirects the metabolism of the heart away from its preferred and most efficient fuel sources, ketones and fatty acids. This explains why heart patients often feel tired before their events and why a diet of liberal amounts of fat and low in glucose is crucial for heart health.

As a result of the sympathetic increase and resulting glycolysis, there is a dramatic increase in lactic acid production in the myocardial cells. This happens in virtually 100 percent of myocardial infarctions, with no coronary artery mechanism required.[7] The increase in lactic acid results in localized acidosis, which makes calcium unable to enter the cells and the cells less able to contract.[8] This inability to contract causes localized edema, hypokinesis or diminished muscle function in the walls of the heart (the hallmark of ischemic disease as seen on echocardiograms and nuclear thallium stress tests)—the build up of lactic acid in the cells and eventually causes necrosis of the tissue, which we call a heart attack.

The localized tissue edema also alters the hemodynamics of the arteries embedded in that section of the heart, causing the pressure that ruptures unstable plaques, which further blocks the artery and worsens the hemodynamics in that area of the heart. This explanation is the only one that answers why plaques rupture, what their role in the myocardial infarction process is, and when and how they should be addressed (i.e., only in the most critical, acute situations). This is the only explanation that accounts for all the observable phenomena associated with heart disease.

So if we want to prevent heart attacks, we must protect our parasympathetic activity, use medicines that support it, and nourish the heart with what it needs. Nourishing our parasympathetic nervous system means dismantling a way of life for which humans are ill suited. This way of life, in my view, is industrial civilization. The known things that nourish our parasympathetic nervous system are contact with nature, loving relations, trust, economic security, and sex—in a sense, a whole new world.

The medicine that supports all aspects of the parasympathetic nervous system is a medicine from the *Strophanthus* plant called ouabain or g-strophanthin. G-strophanthin is an endogenous hormone made in our adrenal cortex from cholesterol—whose production is inhibited by statin drugs—which does two things that are crucial for heart health that no other medicine can do. First, it stimulates the production and liberation of acetylcholine, the main neurotransmitter of the parasympathetic nervous system. Second, and crucially, it converts lactic acid—the main metabolic poison in this process—into pyruvate, one of the main and preferred fuels of the myocardial cells. In other words, it converts a poison into a nutrient. Perhaps this "magic" is why Chinese medicine practitioners say that the kidneys (i.e., the adrenals, where ouabain is made) nourish the heart. In my years of using ouabain in my practice, I have not had a single patient who had a heart attack while taking it. It is truly a gift to the heart.

This understanding of heart disease also leads us to a heart-healthy diet, one that is rich with healthy fats and fat-soluble nutrients and is low in the processed carbohydrates and sugars that practically define industrial civilization.

One might ask why, if heart disease is a disease of industrial civilizations, doesn't the United States have the highest rate of heart disease in the world, or why, within the United States, southern states have a higher rate of heart disease than do the—generally speaking—faster-paced northeastern states. The answer is that, at this point, the entire world has been subjected to industrial civilization and its consequences; it has not confined itself to the American way of life. It is the poorest countries and the poor within the wealthy countries that have the most stress, the most toxic exposure, the worst food, and the fewest opportunities and resources for a healthy lifestyle.

My patients frequently tell me that while they can understand and appreciate the crucial and largely ignored role of the autonomic nervous system in the etiology of heart attacks, they still wonder whether arteriosclerosis plays a role and, if so, whether there is a natural approach to correcting or preventing the development of coronary plaque. Coronary artery sclerosis is a *consequence* of metabolic dysfunction in the heart and can be a deadly consequence if collateral circulation doesn't adequately compensate for the blocked artery. That said, even though collateral circulation can generally compensate for a blockage, this doesn't mean that plaque buildup is a positive development. Arteriosclerosis stiffens and narrows the blood vessels, making blood flow less robust. Here, too, it's important to understand why this happens and how we can prevent it and remediate it if it occurs.

If you think back to how water flows in hydrophilic tubes and how blood flows in vessels, you may remember that there is a protective element built into the system. The exclusion zone, or structured layer, is a thick, viscous, negatively charged coating that lines the inside of the vessel. Pollack chose to call it the exclusion zone because its inherent tendency is to exclude all dissolved substances (solutes) and to repel all other negatively charged particles. This exclusion layer acts as a protection against any corrosive agent that would cause damage to the underlying vessel wall.

If there is a less-than-optimal layer of exclusion zone water, particularly at high-stress areas in the blood vessels, it will result in deterioration of the vessel, which we see pathologically as inflammation. If this inflammation continues unchecked, the body will naturally try to stiffen the weakened artery to allow it to withstand the pressure of the blood flow. It does so by putting a kind of plaster cast made of calcium onto, and even into, the artery. This is what we call plaque. Plaque is the body's compensation mechanism for a weakened artery. To reduce plaque, we need to support the formation of the exclusion zone, reduce the inflammation, and direct calcium to the correct place (the bones).

To support the formation of the exclusion zone, we take advantage of things that have been shown to increase the flow of water through tubes and that provide the energy for the creation of these zones. Pollack's experiments showed that the three most potent energy sources for structuring water are energy from sunlight, the electromagnetic field from the Earth, and the infrared energy that emits from any other living being—the energy from the palms of the hands is a particularly effective way of stimulating blood and water flow. In chapter 11, I talk more about drinking structured water, particularly water with ORME elements in it, to support the structuring of fluids in our bodies. But the simple bottom line is that regular contact with nature, exposure to the sun and the moon, contact with animals, and physical touch with other people is critical to our health.

The second step is to reduce the inflammation in the body and in the blood vessels. More and more cardiologists are recognizing the relationship between an elevated C-reactive protein (a measure of inflammation) and heart disease. While some cardiologists recommend statin drugs to lower the C-reactive protein, a safer approach, and one that addresses the root cause of inflammation, is to deal with hyperinsulinemia, or elevated insulin levels in the blood. Hyperinsulinemia, or metabolic syndrome, occurs when there is a chronic imbalance between the amount of carbohydrates a person consumes and the amount of carbohydrates a person needs. Too many carbohydrates force the body into producing more insulin to lower the blood sugar from diabetic levels. This excess insulin eventually results in obesity (insulin is the hormonal signal to store fat), type II diabetes (a disease characterized by chronically high insulin levels and then eventual resistance to these high levels of insulin, at which point the blood sugar begins to climb), hypertension (insulin causes the body to retain fluid, thus overfilling the circulation and creating high blood pressure), and inflammation. Inflammation in the joints results in arthritis, and in the blood vessels, it results in arteriosclerosis. A sounder approach than the use of toxic anti-inflammatory drugs is to rebalance the diet along the lines of the diets of traditional peoples, the very people who live long, healthy lives with a complete absence of heart disease. I include a sample dietary program in appendix A. Likewise, Sally Fallon's book on traditional diets, *Nourishing Traditions*, should become your constant companion.

The next step in preventing, or in some cases even reversing, arteriosclerosis is to eat a lot of fats, which contain the important fat-soluble vitamin K2. Weston A. Price, the author of *Nutrition and Physical Degeneration* who chronicled the decline in health of indigenous peoples who abandoned their traditional diets in favor of industrial food, was the first to discover the importance of the nutrient he called "Activator X." He found this nutrient, which he claimed was crucial for the proper mineralization of the teeth and bones, to be most abundant in the fat (cream) of cows eating rapidly growing green grass. He produced a centrifuged product from this cream, called butter oil, and used it to treat many ailments, even including some successful remineralizations of teeth with decay and cavities.[9] Modern research has now shown that the function of this "Activator X," now known as vitamin K2, is primarily to direct calcification away from the soft tissues (e.g., arteries) to the bones and teeth where it belongs. Using high doses of modern butter oil or emu oil (which is even higher in this crucial vitamin K2) can, in the context of an otherwise good diet, result in the resolution of calcium deposits in the coronary arteries as inflammation subsides, the exclusion zone is rebuilt, and the protective coating of the plaque is no longer needed.

The final intervention for both prevention and, if present, the treatment of the spectrum of angina, unstable angina, and myocardial infarction is the use of enhanced external counter pulsation (EECP), which is a technology that is successful in helping more than 80 percent of people avoid coronary bypass or stenting.[10] Because it is so successful, EECP challenges the premise that coronary circulation is primarily dependent on the four major coronary arteries. With EECP, the patient lies on a bed, and inflated "balloons" are put on both legs and around the pelvis. The device syncs up the timing of the inflation of the balloons with an EKG so that the balloons are squeezing the legs and pelvis when the heart is in diastole (relaxed). This is done repeatedly for a little over an hour five days a week for seven consecutive weeks. At the end of this time, due to the timed external pressure, the pressurized venous blood essentially creates a new collateral circulation in the heart. Basically, this is an external, nontoxic bypass, but instead of cutting your chest open and inserting a new major vessel that will just become blocked again, EECP does what nature does—it uses flow to create a collateral circulation. In the majority of patients, angina symptoms resolve, heart attacks don't occur, blood vessels become stronger and more flexible, and the resolution lasts for three to seven years, all with the absence of side effects.[11]

CHAPTER EIGHT

Stepping Forth

In the mid-1990s, when I was in my early forties, I began to notice clear signs of a major shift happening in my life. Although my marriage had come to an end, I'd been content and absorbed with living in a small New Hampshire town, managing my practice, studying anthroposophical medicine, and raising my children, when I began to feel restless, as though something that had been working was no longer working. Although I had no real sense yet of why or where I wanted to go next, I began to scratch around for a new place to live.

In particular, I was growing disenchanted with my anthroposophical medical practice. Not only were my patients not getting the results I wanted for them, I was increasingly tired of the jargon in which anthroposophical ideas were frequently discussed. When discussing circulation, for example, we would talk about how it is actually the etheric body, a kind of spiritual force, that causes blood to flow. I was okay with spiritual forces, but I still needed to know how the etheric forces moved the blood. Etheric forces on their own were no longer an acceptable answer for me.

Unfortunately, as I had so often found in my life, anthroposophical medicine didn't offer any kind of road map to answer, or even investigate, these questions. This frustration and my lack of success with my patients led me to the realization that not only was the system of anthroposophical medicine not going to work for me as a lens through which to understand the world, but that no system at all would work for me as a lens through which to understand the world. I had to figure out for myself how I wanted to practice medicine and how I wanted to see, engage with, and understand life. It became clear to me that nobody was ever going to hand me that answer on a silver platter—at least not an answer that I would be satisfied with.

The problem was that having spent a decade doing straight anthroposophical medicine, meaning using the "rules" of anthroposophy to treat people, I found it to be an engaging exercise for me, but the results were less than optimal for my patients. I'm still not really sure why it doesn't work as well as it "should," but it doesn't—that was my experience. As a result, I could no longer just do anthroposophy as my primary medical therapy. I had to find some other way to incorporate the big picture issues that I was aware of and that I wanted my practice to be grounded in.

Although this was disconcerting to some extent, it also freed me to ask the important question of "what next?" This openness to a new way of seeing medicine, to a new way of understanding life's deepest processes, to a new place to live, to new people in my life was a little frightening but mostly familiar for me. I already felt at home in the uncertainty of life. My comfort in this place of uncertainty allowed me to meet two of the most important people who have ever walked into my life.

I had been studying food as medicine, the ecology of food, and everything food-related since at least my late teens. Over the years, I'd spent time at the Hippocrates Health Institute, studied macrobiotics with Michio Kushi in Boston, and was an original member of the first CSA in the United States. I had tried on myself and my patients just about every diet there was. And while I always remained fascinated with the work of Weston A. Price, I found it impossible to go from his writing to figuring out how and what to eat at the end of the twentieth century, after so much had changed from the world he'd studied. He was clear about the importance of diet and food grown from healthy soil, but he wasn't specific about what a modern person should eat to reflect the traditional diets he'd studied.

Then I read an interview with Sally Fallon about her recently published book, *Nourishing Traditions*. By the time I finished reading the interview, I was both excited to meet this woman and irritated that after all the time I'd spent studying food, she clearly knew more about it than I did. I immediately called her, asked her how she knew what she knew, and invited her to do her first public seminar at my practice in New Hampshire. At that meeting, we decided to collaborate on a book on food, medicine, and movement, which eventually became *The Fourfold Path to Healing*, coauthored along with Jaimen McMillen, a friend of mine who developed the movement art called spatial dynamics.

As we worked on the book over the next few years, I supported Sally in starting The Weston A. Price Foundation, now a significant voice for the traditional foods movement worldwide. With her vast knowledge, Sally revolutionized the natural foods movement in the United States. She is largely responsible for the availability of foods like broth, butter, ghee, coconut oil, fermented vegetables, and kombucha. And the social movement that developed alongside *Nourishing Traditions* and The Weston A. Price Foundation is as responsible as any for the rejuvenation of small farms and food businesses.

It was over the past fifteen years working with Sally, doing annual Fourfold conferences, writing *The Fourfold Path to Healing* and then *The Nourishing Traditions Book of Baby and Childcare*, and giving annual talks at The Weston A. Price Foundation's Wise Traditions conference that I began to find my voice. Some say that life can only unfold through our connections with others. It was, to a great degree, through my connection with and support from Sally Fallon that I was able to take a significant step in the unfolding of my professional life.

And then—extremely uncharacteristically for me—I walked into a donut shop in Fair Oaks, California, on August 11, 1998. I was in Fair Oaks to attend what would be my final anthroposophic event, at a time when it was becoming more and more clear that I needed to find my own way. I had been invited to give a talk on the healing aspects of fairy tales, one of those things that all anthroposophical doctors must know, particularly the esoteric significance behind the story. But I was also there to hang out with a good friend of mine who had also been invited to speak. When I'd arrived, I'd learned that my friend had canceled at the last minute.

Feeling stuck and frustrated on a hundred-plus-degree day, I attended some of the talks, gave my workshop, and waited to go back home. There was a theatrical performance that I just could not sit through. I left early, annoyed and hungry, and inexplicably stopped at the donut shop on my way home. I ordered a frozen yogurt, turned around in line, and saw this person whom I instantly knew—but what word can one even use that can capture a moment like this?—was my soul mate. I knew within minutes that while she might not agree, for my part at least, I was going to do everything I could to never be without this woman for the rest of my life.

For those of you who have experienced such a moment, you know that words simply cannot capture what some would call a feeling but which in reality is larger than that. It was the closest I'd ever come to knowing something, really knowing it, as opposed to thinking or even feeling something, in my entire life. Describing what I saw doesn't do justice to the experience. It wasn't just that she was the most beautiful woman I had ever seen, though she was. It wasn't her magical smile, though she has that. It wasn't a kind of grace and tenderness that one rarely meets, though she has that, too. It was that I sensed for the first time that I had met my other half, my partner in life. It was the taking of another's hand and acknowledging, with an almost unfathomable sense of relief, that I was alone no more.

Five days later, en route home to New Hampshire from California, I laid out my plans for how we could make this work, get married, and figure out a way for me to eventually move to San Francisco, her beloved home. It was all crazy, but I was very clear—and she would choose for herself, of course—that I was going to make this happen. As Lynda has said, it was like choosing when there is really no choice. Our way forward together was a *fait accompli*.

As all this was happening in my life, I felt it was time for the next canoe trip, a trip that my heart used to remind me not to forget about my old internal friend.

During our first few years together, Lynda and I lived in New Hampshire until we could figure out how to get us both to San Francisco. We bought a beautiful wooden canoe, spent many evenings canoeing on the many small lakes of southern New Hampshire, and took a few short canoe camping trips. Then when it was time, we moved to San Francisco to establish a new home and new practice for me. It was an exciting time for us, with many new things to explore, and on my agenda was a trip to the one major canoeing destination in North America that I had not yet seen—the Boundary Waters Canoe Area Wilderness in northern Minnesota. A vast series of lakes and small islands with almost no roads or other access, the wilderness area is the crown jewel of canoe camping.

I organized the trip, made the arrangements, and then Lynda and I flew to Ely, Minnesota, for our week in the wilderness. Lynda was a little unsure but a good sport and willing participant. The first day and first night were composed of gorgeous, clear waters; ancient paintings on vast boulders that framed a majestic lake; and camping on the shore under brilliant stars in a pitch black sky.

The next day, however, it took us way too long to find our campsite. We hurried to set up camp. I was chopping wood when my heart set off running with SVT. In the previous few years, it had been happening more and more, between two and ten times a week, often with no significant exertion, but by simply being a little anxious—before giving a public talk before a large audience, for example. Like water flowing down a riverbed, the more the water travels down a certain channel over time, the deeper and more grooved the channel becomes, making it easier for the water to more regularly travel this route. And I had been having greater and greater difficulty converting the rhythm back to normal. I began taking beta-blockers with me on outings that involved significant stress or exertion.

Deep in the wilderness, with nobody but Lynda in sight, I became anxious. I knew it was a "mistake" to get anxious because anxiety would only exacerbate the condition, but I could hardly have helped it. I took a beta-blocker and did all the things I usually do to coax my heart back to its regular rhythm: lying down with my knees above my head, performing the Valsalva maneuver, rubbing the carotid artery, taking deep breaths—all things known to ease SVT. It didn't stop. It was the first time I couldn't bring it back under control. I was worried about it but was also worried about setting up camp before it got dark, so I persisted with my camp tasks, also a mistake.

Finally, after an hour at a rate of two hundred beats per minute, I lay down on the forest floor to try to calm my heart. Assaulted by mosquitoes, I moved into the tent, where I lay first on my sleeping bag, then on Lynda's lap, and focused completely on trying calm my racing heart. My anxiety, intensified by a sense of claustrophobia, turned into dread, making it harder to control my body and increasingly scary. Hours passed. I lay still, meditated, whatever, but nothing worked. Lynda read from a book of Native American stories and poems. Still nothing worked. Around 2 a.m., I started to cough. I grew short of breath, coughing up frothy sputum. I was going into heart failure on a remote island in northern Minnesota. I was going to die, I thought, within hours.

I had sometimes wondered what it might feel like, or what I might think, at such a time. But I didn't experience any profound insights. All I thought was, "I want to breathe." But I also had a decision to make: Should I take another beta-blocker to see if it could break the rhythm, knowing that it might worsen the heart failure? I took the next pill and almost immediately fell asleep in Lynda's arms.

I woke up an hour later and whispered to Lynda, "It broke." Lynda replied—and I can hear her saying this as if it were yesterday—"Don't move." I lay dozing until daylight, my breathing gradually recovering. I was exhausted.

———◆———

Lynda decided to paddle for help. She was not as strong a paddler as I, and she had never paddled solo, but she canoed across a strong current to the nearest island. She beached the canoe, wedged it into some rocks, and scaled a steep incline, terrified of falling backward down the slope and into the water. Once on the island, she found a canoe "parked" on a beach and discovered a middle-aged couple having breakfast nearby. In fairly atypical behavior for Lynda, she burst into tears and recounted our story.

These wonderful people helped her catch her breath, ferried Lynda and our canoe back to our island, and discovered the state I was in. They paddled for three hours to one of the only points in the lakes that could be traversed by motorboats. There they waited until a passing boat stopped and radioed for help. This couple was able to precisely identify our island on a map, allowing a small team of rescuers to arrive by water plane and fly us out to Ely.

By then, my heart rate had returned to its normal rhythm and my breathing had improved, although I was exhausted in a way I have never experienced before. But I knew at that point that I would be OK, and so I resisted going to the hospital. Lynda asserted that she was "making the decisions now," and so off we went.

The ER doctor in Ely thought, incorrectly, that I'd had a mild heart attack brought on by the stress of the prolonged rapid heart rate and insisted on sending me by ambulance to the regional cardiac hospital in Duluth. There, I was seen by a friendly cardiologist whom I was able to persuade that the best course of action was to observe my condition with no interventions. I was released the next day with instructions to take regular beta-blockers until I returned home and to see an electrophysiologist to ablate (laser out) an extra pathway and stop this from ever happening again. Lynda, who was emboldened by hearing opinions other than my own on what our options were and who knew how the SVT was interfering with my life, "loved" me into having the ablation a few months later. (Other possible words for it would be "forced," or "cajoled," because I was—admittedly—stubborn about being a patient.) In the ten years since, I have not experienced the symptoms.

Our trip to the Boundary Waters was, in the end, humbling and revealing, and it provoked a great deal of soul-searching for me. It softened my sometimes overly strident stance against technology in medicine. And it launched me into the next phase of my understanding of the heart. It was the ablation that drove me to investigate what really happens in the heart and why the heart gets sick. Strangely enough, this path led to water, and the movement of water, and the relevance of love in maintaining the health of the heart. Not unlike that last canoe trip.

CHAPTER NINE

Treating the Heart

For about twelve years now, I have been prescribing a new approach to my patients who suffer angina, unstable angina, and myocardial infarction. These patients have come to me at all stages of sickness and health. Some have come because of a family history of heart disease and want a preventative approach. Others come because of the onset of chest pain with or without exertion. And some come saying they have "high cholesterol" and are told they need a lifelong regimen of drugs that they don't want to take—either because they tried them and couldn't tolerate the side effects or because it just didn't feel right for them.

But the majority of my heart patients come after having suffered a heart attack, often after having had bypass surgery or multiple stents placed. These patients often feel better after the surgery, which isn't surprising—bypasses and stents relieve symptoms. These patients are also keenly aware of three things. One is that they "haven't been the same" since the heart attack and the procedures they've undergone. Often this experience is vague: Their energy is not the same, they feel less vitality, or something simply feels missing. They often chalk it up to aging, but the feeling is nevertheless clear and unsettling to most of these people.

The second experience is similar but has more to do with side effects of the medications that heart disease patients are placed on after a heart attack or angina episode. The statin drugs leave them feeling weak, unable to do their usual activities; their memory feels less sharp; and they experience an unfamiliar lethargy. The beta-blockers also leave them tired, often with erectile dysfunction and a new, unfamiliar depression. The blood-thinning medicines, usually Plavix and aspirin, leave them bruised and anxious about the risk of potentially fatal internal bleeding. My patients are savvy, informed people; they are well aware of the controversies surrounding the use of this cocktail of medicines long term. Like many of us, they are asking a simple and straightforward question: Isn't there a way to treat my condition that makes me stronger and healthier rather than in a state of progressive deterioration? It is this question, more than anything else, that leads people to my door.

I tell many of my patients that I believe in the anvil theory of medicine: Say you are not prone to headaches. Then one day you are walking down the street and an anvil falls on your head. After that, you have daily headaches. It's probably from the anvil.

Some doctors don't believe in the anvil theory. A colleague of mine was an air force flight surgeon. At his yearly physical, he was told he had high cholesterol and that he needed to take the statin drug Lipitor if he wanted to keep flying. A few weeks after starting the Lipitor, he experienced a bout of amnesia while flying. He asked his doctor if was from the Lipitor and was told no. Suspicious, my colleague stopped the drug and didn't experience amnesia again. A year later, after he'd started the drug again so that he could continue flying, he experienced another bout of amnesia. His doctor again insisted that it was *not* caused by the

Lipitor. My colleague began to research the connection himself, set up a website to compile stories from other patients on statin drugs, and eventually wrote a book called *Lipitor: Thief of Memory*, detailing the mechanisms whereby statin drugs impede memory, inspired by the stories of thousands of people who had suffered the same symptoms. Besides pointing out one of the dangers of statin drugs, the point of this story is that a lot of doctors either don't believe in the anvil or, even if they do, don't bother to take the time to ask their patients the right questions or even listen to their story. As a doctor, this is a mistake I never want to make.

So when a heart patient—or any patient, for that matter—comes to me, I always start with the question: "So what happened to you?" Another way to ask this is: "Tell me about when you last felt well, and then bring me up to present time." In other words, tell me your story. What is most compelling to me about this approach is that patients, in general, and heart patients, in particular, don't only tell me about the anvil events; they have an intuitive sense that the illness of their heart is related to other things—the losses, the stresses, the loves, and the challenges in their lives.

I encourage them to include things they may have been told have nothing to do with heart disease. Heart disease, as we have learned, is not just the plaque in the coronary arteries. I am looking and listening for the events in their lives that have caused a suppression of their parasympathetic nervous system—their sense of well-being in their lives. So we start the therapy with their story and an emphasis on certain events in their lives. This, in itself, is often cathartic and a first step toward healing an ailing heart.

When a patient is telling his or her story, I never offer any advice or venture an opinion on whether a given event "caused" their heart disease. I have too much respect for the inner process going on in a person's life to intervene in this way. It is simply, and powerfully, a telling—or, possibly, a retelling—of one's life. The telling of the story is not to be commented on or corrected in any way. Done well, it is perhaps the most therapeutic step toward recovery that many people ever experience—to be listened to with empathy. In our culture, this is actually a revolutionary way to practice medicine, to begin by listening deeply to a patient. It is always the place to start. And hopefully, in telling her story, the patient finds her own anvil and, with this revelation, can begin to make some changes in her life.

Then we move on: What do you eat? When and how do you sleep? What do you do most of the day? How do you move your body? Do you sit most of the time? Whom do you spend your time with? How are your family relationships and all the other details that make up a life?

In a patient's answers to these questions, I am listening for the heart. There is evidence that our core personality, our core outlook, our core tendencies reside in our physical heart (see chapter 12). I want to understand the heart of the person sitting with me, and I want him to hear himself relate the details of how he lives. Before our treatment, maybe his diet was haphazard, he spent most of the time not moving his body, and he was often anxious and depressed about his illness and other things in his life, if maybe only subtly. As our treatment goes on, we revisit the story and the details as we continue to learn and understand how his heart is doing.

Then I do a physical exam to get a sense of the integrity of the physical body. How is the blood pressure? How is the pulse—not just the rate, but the character and strength and integrity of the pulse? Is the pulse weak and timid, strong and bounding, erratic and jumpy? This helps me understand the essence of the patient asking for my help. I look at the eyes, the irises, the tongue. Is this a swollen, moist person or a dry, more withered type? I can see and understand this by studying the tongue.

I listen to the heart and lungs. In particular, I am listening to the quality of two distinct heart sounds. When you listen to the heart, there are at least five distinct "sites" where you can listen. Each of these sites accentuates or diminishes one of the two heart sounds. Starting at the upper border of the left side of the sternum and working down the left sternal border and over to the apex of the heart, you hear the different intensity (loudness) of the two sounds. In a healthy person, very near the bottom of the left side of the sternum, the two sounds are of equal intensity; this equal intensity suggests that the sympathetic nervous system influences from above (the head, the nervous system) are in balance with the parasympathetic nervous system influences from below (the metabolism) in this central meeting space of the heart. This is as it should be.

We are striving for balance. The sympathetic and parasympathetic forces should meet in intensity at the left lower border of the heart. It is here that the two heart sounds should be equal in intensity. One hears "lub-dub." At the top of the left sternal border one hears "LUB-dub" where the first, or nervous system, sound is accentuated. At the apex, or directly under the nipple line, one should hear something like "lub-DUB" where the second, or metabolic sound, is loudest and most intense.

In a balanced autonomic nervous system, the heart sounds should be equal in intensity at the lower left sternal border. When they are not balanced here, it tells me which part of the autonomic nervous system is predominant. In the majority of people with heart disease, the sympathetic nervous system is predominant. This is heard in a "LUB-dub" sound even all the way over to the apex of the heart. Over time, with therapy, we can observe if it starts to correct itself.

From there, I feel the abdomen. In particular, I am looking for swollen organs, especially a congested liver, which suggests that the metabolism is burdened and sick. Finally, I examine the legs to look for signs of swollen or congested veins (where blood circulation starts, as described in chapter 2). I look for the presence of edema, or swelling in the legs, an indication that the circulation is compromised. Having listened to the story and completed an exam, I have a sense not only of a patient's life and the integrity of his or her physical body, but of how well balanced the autonomic nervous system is, as well as the quality of the person's circulation.

Then we move on to testing. Generally speaking, I am more of a minimalist than most. The most important tests I look at when evaluating a person with known or suspected heart issues are the HgbA1c, the hsCRP, and a stress echo. The test for HgbA1c, also known as glycosylated hemoglobin, tells us the average blood sugar over approximately the past eight weeks, providing the most accurate assessment of blood sugar and the existence of diabetes, prediabetes, and overall metabolic control. A person with a consistent HgbA1c result of less than 5.3 will typically have no evidence of heart disease of any kind. This level suggests tight blood sugar control, low insulin levels, minimal or no inflammation, and—crucially—no small vessel (capillary) disease. The higher the A1c, the more likely we are to find these issues. A result over 6.2 strongly suggests significant plaque, metabolic dysfunction of the heart, autonomic imbalance, and small vessel disease. This we can then address with a metabolic restoration program of diet and movement.

HsCRP—high-sensitivity C-reactive protein—is a marker for inflammation, usually related to the A1c. This number tells us about inflammation in the blood vessels. An ideal value is less than 0.5. When it approaches or exceeds 3, significant inflammation is typical. At this level, one begins to see signs of plaque development and small blood vessel disease. This can also be addressed with a prescribed diet and movement program.

Finally, the stress echo assesses the heart's ability to move under the stress of physical exertion. The heart needs to move and be flexible. A stiff or inflexible area of the heart, which cardiologists interpret as a blocked artery, means that all of the metabolic processes that result in normal muscle movement are impaired in that area of the heart. Blood flow through both large vessels (coronary arteries) and small vessels (capillaries) impacts the integrity of the myocardial cells and their ability to metabolize fuel and get rid of waste products, and therefore blood flow also influences the movements of the heart as a whole, which is what the stress echo evaluates. Part of the heart's ability to move in a healthy way is due to the influence of the metabolism, whether or not inflammation is present and if the autonomic nervous system is in balance. If we see impaired movement of the heart, we assess whether our heart therapy can restore a normal movement pattern in the heart.

Once I've listened to a patient's story, completed a physical exam, and looked at the results of any tests, we can move on to treatment, which consists of retelling one's story, changing one's diet, introducing certain kinds of movement, medicines (especially *Strophanthus* extract or g-strophanthin/ouabain), and EECP.

I outlined the details of some of these interventions in chapter 7, including a *Nourishing Traditions*–type diet of liberal fats and low carbohydrates, which is especially effective in treating the metabolic defects reflected in the elevated A1c and hsCRP levels underlying heart disease. For movement, the basic plan is thirty minutes per day of barefoot walking when possible, especially on a beach for those who live near the ocean, or thirty minutes per day of vigorous outside walking if barefoot walking is not possible. Thirty minutes per day of walking on a treadmill is the third best option.

The benefits of barefoot walking, or "earthing," are based on the same influences that make water move (see chapter 2). Making our water (i.e., blood) move is an important component of healthy circulation, of which the heart is a part. Increased blood flow means increased metabolism, which translates to a restoration of the health of the heart as a muscle. Vigorous barefoot walking is a key to improving blood flow and overall circulation.

The other movement strategy that is important for improving muscle metabolism, including the heart, and encouraging new small blood vessel formation is a once-per-week high-intensity strength training, such as Ken Hutchens's SuperSlow program, although any kind of similar high-intensity training will work. This type of training encourages muscle growth and the formation of the new blood vessels to support this muscle growth. It is best done under the supervision of a trainer who is skilled in helping people develop a strength-training program.

The medicine program is generally simple and straightforward. G-strophanthin is taken at a dose of three milligrams two to three times per day, usually first thing in the morning and in the evening. *Strophanthus* is also available as an extract, in which case it should be used at five to twenty drops three times per day, before meals. The medicine should be kept in the mouth for one minute before swallowing because it is best absorbed through the oral mucosa. (You could break open the capsule and put pure g-strophanthin powder in your mouth for a minute, and people have done this, but it is unbelievably bitter, so most people only try this once.)

The dose is titrated up or down depending on a person's reaction to it. This is very important and why it is best to work with a doctor who is experienced in using g-strophanthin (or *Strophanthus* extract). There are rarely negative effects, but each person must find their optimal dose regardless of whether they're using capsules or liquid extracts. The effect we are looking for is a sense of relief of the symptoms. This can be a steadier rhythm, less pain, more stamina, less psychological tension, better sleep, and overall better function. After some months, we look to see if the stress echo has improved, suggesting overall better metabolic function in the heart. Once we've found the most effective dose, I generally keep my patients on this dose indefinitely, often for the rest of their lives.

G-strophanthin is not yet—or not anymore, depending on how you look at it—widely available. Many years ago, g-strophanthin was sold as a prescription medication in capsule form in the United States. A few decades ago, it vanished completely in the United States but continued to be sold over the counter in Germany and Europe. Currently, the only source I know of in the world that makes the pure g-strophanthin capsules is a compounding pharmacy in Germany by prescription only. And the only source I know of for the extract is a company in Brazil that makes its extract from *Strophanthus* seeds; it contains the active ingredient g-strophanthin. While it is a safe medicine, it is crucial that *Strophanthus* be used only under the care of a health practitioner who is well versed in its use. There is currently a worldwide project to bring a new, improved, safe, and legal form of g-strophanthin at least to the European market, but it is years, maybe decades, away.

The only other routine medicine I use is six capsules of emu oil per day, which, due to the particular fats and high amounts of vitamin K2, helps to soften the blood vessels. In some cases, I have seen plaque that had built up in the coronary arteries dissolve slightly.

Finally, if possible, we do a seven-week course of EECP to reduce chest pains, improve functional capacity, and restore normal small blood vessel or collateral circulation. Usually this seven-week course of treatment is effective for relieving angina and improving the functional capacity of the patient. Overall blood flow improves, the blood flow in the heart is more robust, and stamina improves greatly. EECP protects the heart from damage and generally it need not be repeated for five to seven years.

This is the basic outline of the program. We modify the approach depending on the particular needs and symptoms of the patient. Some patients need help with liver congestion; others may need more guidance in relaxation techniques. Hopefully, at some point soon, more physicians will become fluent in strategies for metabolic restoration of their patients and, as follows, participate in real healing for people with heart troubles. It is a missing skill that is urgently needed.

So how does all this work in reality? One of the first patients I treated with *Strophanthus* came to me about twelve years ago. He was a diabetic Russian immigrant in his midseventies who had spent many years in a Siberian camp under the old Soviet empire. He was freed following the collapse of the Soviet Union and came to the United States to live out the rest of his life. His initial complaint to me was severe shortness of breath and chest pain with little exertion. Although his main joy in life was cross-country skiing, when I first met him he couldn't even walk to his mailbox without fatigue and chest pain.

At the time, my main interventions were diet and Strodival (a form of g-strophanthin that is no longer available). After two months of this regimen, his diabetes resolved, and he was able to resume cross-country skiing. This continued with very few other interventions for seven years, at which time—in his eighties—he began to slow down. He told me at every appointment that he needed to feel free—no surprise there, after what he had been through—and he said this feeling only came when he was skiing. He felt that the diet and the *Strophanthus* had given him his life back.

When people are under stress, either short- or long-term, they often begin to experience heart symptoms, including such things as tachycardia (fast heart rate), arrhythmias (often felt as skipped beats), anxiety, or chest pains. Some of these symptoms are indicative of or lead to further heart problems. It's critical to resolve this physiological stress state at an early stage to prevent the development of further issues down the road.

One patient, who was in a dominant sympathetic nervous system state when she came to see me, soon wrote to me: "I wanted to drop you a quick note to thank you for the addition of the ouabain in my life. I have already experienced so many positive changes in my health and life. I have experienced only one episode of bad dreams and racing heart since beginning the ouabain, instead of three or four times per week. I sleep soundly throughout the night. I used to get up once or twice to urinate.

I am calmer throughout the day and have a more positive disposition. I have greater exercise tolerance with a great steady heart rate. My resting heart rate has gone down from the 80s to the 60s. I rarely hear my heart beating in my head or ears. I am so appreciative that you, as an MD, have chosen to practice true 'integrative' medicine, with a focus on the most effective natural options available."

Hidden within these kind words is a picture of the autonomic nervous system imbalance that underlies heart issues. Before beginning a regimen of g-strophanthin, she was in a dominant sympathetic nervous system state. This was quickly and directly resolved with the simple addition of the ouabain without any changes to her lifestyle. Of course, g-strophanthin is most effective in concert with the other therapies, but I do have patients who don't want to do anything about their diet or physical activity; they only opt for the g-strophanthin. Amazingly, especially when the main source of their heart disease is autonomic imbalance, which it often is, they often experience quick and sometimes profound relief.

Another letter came in from a gentleman in his midsixties who had already had his first stent replaced with a second at the time he first came to me. A spiritual person, this man worried about the impact that toxic prescription drugs would have on his physical, mental, and spiritual well-being, so he was looking for another way.

"One morning I woke up and felt a pressure on my chest, so I got out of bed and stood up to take the pressure off my chest. After three hours, sitting in a chair and feeling that something was not right, my wife took me to the hospital. Confronted with the fact of a heart attack I had few choices. Perhaps the stent and all the 'medicines' saved my life. In the initial period afterwards, I tried to eat a low-fat diet. That, with the drugs that had been prescribed for me, would have been the end of me.... [With a] diet high in fat, cholesterol, and Himalayan salt, and also, *Strophanthus*, the response to these changes was immediate. I felt like a human being again. It just kept getting better as we discontinued the prescription drugs. The *Strophanthus* did the impossible: It opened my heart, my feeling self, up! Also, it lowered my blood pressure. I cannot understand how a homeopathic remedy can do this! A little later, I asked: What more could I do to change my life so that I would not get another heart attack. My wife and I began a low-carb diet. We both lost twenty pounds, which did not come back, and felt in control of our lives for once. While regular medicine treated my heart problems with massive force, [you] treated me with understanding. Which do you think I prefer?"

What is particularly compelling about this man's testimonial is what he writes about opening up his heart and feeling his "self" again. As we will see in chapter 12, the physical heart is the repository of that which we call the self. The experience of a real heart therapy is to regain, or even "improve," on one's capacity for opening the heart and finding one's true self. Many years later, this man continues to have no cardiac symptoms, is on no prescription medicines, and needed no further cardiac interventions.

CHAPTER TEN

The Cosmic Heart

We have come to a transition point. Up to now, I have mainly concerned myself with the human heart. We have explored circulation, the form and function of the human heart, and the causes and treatments of the most common type of heart disease—the number one cause of death worldwide.[1] Why not stop there?

I can't stop there because my goal has always been to write a book that understands, as deeply as possible, the causes of illness. There is no way to heal without understanding cause. And it has become increasingly clear to me over my career that to decontextualize illness from its social, economic, political, and personal context is a gross error. Illnesses are *defined* in cultural and social context. A person we might label as the victim of psychosis, delusions, or schizophrenia in the United States might be revered as a village shaman or holy man in another culture. The ailments we treat with billions of dollars of questionable heart medications and chest-cracking surgeries might be considered the consequence of spiritual or personal crisis for many of the world's people. While we might dismiss this "primitive" way of seeing the world, it's not as though our industrialized medical system offers a medical slam dunk. Where certain communicable disease rates have dropped in the United States, chronic disease rates are on the rise. Any honest doctor must concern theirself with the larger context of the illnesses of their patients.

For example, 8 percent of prisoners worldwide are African American men imprisoned in the United States.[2] Might this be a larger health problem for African American communities than cholesterol levels? The main cause of death for children living in the Gaza Strip is war-related trauma.[3] Might this be a comparable, or larger, public health issue than whether they are vaccinated against measles? Every drop of mother's milk, human or animal, on the entire planet is contaminated with toxic and carcinogenic chemicals. Are we to believe that group B strep in the birth canal or hepatitis B injections within hours after the birth are a more important intervention than a public health initiative to make sure these types of chemicals never show up in our mothers' milk?

I realize I'm making an apples-to-oranges comparison, but the salient point is that these and hundreds of other examples I could offer never show up at cardiology conferences, medical journals, or even in the writings of holistic health practitioners. But they need to. We need to begin to draw these connections. I know this because I realized, as I was thinking about and working on this book, that I couldn't write a book exploring the roots of illness—*without exploring the roots of illness.*

The roots of illness lie in the world around us. These roots include how we treat the world and the social, economic, political system we are "swimming" in. The world around us, including our perception of it, affects us as much as coral reefs are affected by the health of the world's oceans. This is a crucial point and my thesis: Understanding "the cosmic heart" is the key to unlocking the larger context that we humans currently find ourselves in. It provides a blueprint for the healthier, happier, more joyous world that we know in our hearts is possible.

There is that word again. Heart. And if the idea of a "cosmic heart" seems too woo-woo, consider the language that has developed around our heart. Why do we say, "I know in my heart that it's possible." Why do we associate the heart with love, romance, courage, heroism—if it's only a muscle that pumps blood? Why do we talk about someone having a heart of gold?

Science can provide some tools to help us understand the heart and what ails it. But science alone is inadequate. And, in this sense, we've begun to travel a dangerous path of putting all of our trust, all of our faith and belief, in science—as the only legitimate way of knowing. If science is something akin to "the knowledge about or study of the natural world based on facts learned through experiments and observation,"[4] how does it account for something like love? I know for a fact that love exists—I would hope that anyone with a child, or a parent, or possibly a spouse would, too—but I don't have a clue how science would prove it. Exploring the cosmic heart is a step—and I believe a crucial step—in breaking what I would call the spell of the cult of science that threatens to kill us all.

While I was in medical school, I had the opportunity to attend a lecture on anthroposophy given by an anthroposophist, astronomer, and physicist named Norman Davidson. The first thing out of Davidson's mouth, in one of the first lectures about anthroposophy I ever heard, was that "the single most important concept that you must deeply understand if you are to know, really know, anything about the stars, or planets, or yourself, is to understand that the Earth is still and the sun, planets, and stars rotate around us, not the other way around." As people stood up and headed for the exit, I thought, "I must be in the right place."

We learn in school that our solar system is made up of a "fixed" sun around which orbit, at various distances from this sun, the planets of our solar system. We learn that the pathways are not exactly circular orbits but more like ellipses. (This is not actually true; the sun spirals through space and the planets are pulled in a spiral pathway around this spiraling sun). We learn that the Earth is traveling about 11,000 miles per hour in this elliptical pathway and it is spinning on its tilted axis—tilted at 23 degrees from vertical—at approximately 1,000 miles per hour.

Imagine trying to convince an audience of people who have never gone to school, who spend most of their days outside engaged with the natural world through farming, hunting, or gathering, that they are hurtling through space at enormous speeds, while spinning like a giant top. Try to tell them that the sun they see rising every morning in the east and setting every night in the west is not actually moving, but that—on the contrary—we are the ones who are moving. Good luck with that talk!

Recently I gave a talk in front of about 500 people, about 98 percent of whom (I asked) had college or advanced degrees. I asked how many knew who came up with the idea that the Earth goes around the sun and not vice versa. Most, though not all, people in the audience raised their hands. It was Copernicus, of course, the sixteenth-century Polish astronomer who wrote the original treatise on this heliocentric theory of planetary movement.

Then I asked how many people in the audience knew what simple observation we can all make that can only be explained by the heliocentric theory. Amazingly—and I say amazingly because the transition from the geocentric model to the heliocentric model was such a massive turning point in the history of humanity with repercussions that echo, indeed dominate, to this day that you would think that anyone who'd ever gone to school would know this fact—only one person raised his hand. He explained that there is observable retrograde movement of the planets, which could not occur if they were circling around the Earth. In fact, one of the reasons that planets—from the Greek word for "wanderer"—are called planets is because of what a perplexing phenomenon this was in the geocentric model.

Even for those of us who don't understand why the heliocentric paradigm is correct—and, based on that experience in my lecture, I'd suggest that a startlingly small number of us do—many of us westerners would still cite science as a superior way of knowing compared to more "primitive" ways of knowing. So let's make a report card to evaluate performance and compare characteristics determined by (or at least associated with) each paradigm.

People who believe(d) in the geocentric model generally:

- Lived in sustainable societies for thousands of years.
- Often improved the health of the ecosphere, including plant, animal, and soil life, the more they engaged with it.
- Did not cause widespread extinction of other animals or plants.
- Had no toxic or carcinogenic chemicals in their breast milk.
- Had no heart attacks—ever.

People who believe(d) in the heliocentric model generally:

- Live in unsustainable societies, compounding the depletion of stored resources each year.
- Degrade the health of the biosphere to such an extent that it results in massive extinctions and widespread desertification.
- Have numerous toxic and carcinogenic chemicals in their breast milk (or bodies, as the case may be).
- Are at high risk of suffering a heart attack.

I am aware that correlation is not causation. Nor am I claiming that belief in the heliocentric model has caused the above things to happen. At the same time, it's important to acknowledge that the shift from the geocentric to the heliocentric paradigm was a massive turning point in the way humans inter-act with the world around us—and from this turning point, so many catastrophes have followed.

With this as an introduction, we can now move on to explore what I mean when I use the expression "cosmic heart." What do I mean by this? The forces, power, and activities of the human heart are the same forces, powers, and processes—or are in some way connected—with the forces, powers, and processes in the wider cosmos. Consider this as a place to start: We have already seen that the form of the heart can be visualized as a chestahe-dron that sits in a cube at an angle of slightly more than 36 degrees to the left of center. This is the same angle at which the human heart sits in the chest. And this is the approximate Cen-tigrade temperature (if slightly higher) of normothermia, or normal human body temperature. We refer to a compassionate person as warm-hearted; maybe our human warmth actually comes from the heart.

The human heart is not simply embedded in the rhythms of the cosmos. Research from the HeartMath Institute, a non-profit dedicated to bringing people's physical, mental, and emotional systems into alignment with the heart's intuitive guidance, has shown that the heart acts like a conductor in the body and other organs entrain on or pick up rhythms from it.[5] In this way, these different organs are able to integrate into one whole, living system.

A human being takes an average of 25,920 breaths per day (average 18 breaths/minute × 60 minutes × 24 hours); it takes the sun about the same number of years to traverse the twelve signs of the zodiac—the so-called Platonic year. The sun travels one degree of the zodiac every seventy-two years—the average approximate length of the human life. In these seventy-two years, there are about 26,000 days—the approximate number of breaths in a day or the time for the sun to make one complete cycle of the celestial world. Finally, between each cycle of inha-lation and exhalation, there is a slight pause that helps prevent hyperventilation. There is a similar pause in the cycle of the year. At the solstice, the sun "rests" for a moment, and then swings back the other way (at least as observed by the human being from Earth).

These calculations originate from a geocentric view of the universe—what you can see and experience if you stand at the center of the universe, looking up to the heavens above—not from a heliocentric view of the universe, where scientists might quibble with some of the numbers.[6] But this is the perspective that allowed traditional people who were intimately familiar with these rhythms to find their way home, or afield, by observing the stars. They knew how to plant, tend to, and harvest crops and understand the unique pattern of seasonal and celestial events that each individual is born into. And it's a perspective that Steiner emphasized over and over as the archetypal, or "perfect," rhythm. A human being—and her rhythmic system of the heart and lungs (pulse and breathing)—exists in the ratio of 1:4, the "creation" rhythm (i.e., bowing to the four directions or the composition of a perfect square).

Most importantly, this perspective gave people a sense of place in the vast universe in which they found themselves. It offered a foundation of rootedness, perspective, and uniqueness for each individual being. A view of the heavens varies in every place, whether one is looking up from present-day Nebraska or Sri Lanka. This is a worldview that truly values a person's place and suggests that everything else in the world also has a unique place and role in the cosmic order. It is a fundamentally qualitative view of the world. It is also a perspective of security and trust. Geocentric people felt or knew they could trust what they saw and experienced. They knew they were tied to a place and other beings within a cosmic order that they could largely understand, use, and rely on. It is out of this sense of familiarity, trust, and uniqueness that love and care can arise. And although it's an ideal, it's an ideal that represents harmony, toward which we should strive.

You won't care for your piece of land if, when you "use it up," you just move on to the next similar such field to grow the same crops. We don't love all women equally; we love *our* mother or our soul mate. We don't love and care for all children equally. Through experience, trust, and connection, we love *our* child or children. We don't all love land equally; we love the land we have a connection to, that which provides us with what we need to maintain life.

Heliocentricism teaches us to distrust our own experience. We learn that we are hurtling through space, spinning like a top. Nothing that happens in the wider cosmos, to or from the other planets in our solar system, has any relation to us. Our place is not unique in any real sense. We study what happens to trees as a result of certain phenomena, as if all trees in a forest, or plants in a field, or cows on a dairy farm, or rats in a laboratory are identical. And what about fellow humans? If they happen to be poor, unschooled, or live on rich mineral or oil deposits, their uniqueness is not so crucial. How unique can anyone be when many of us take vows of "to death do we part" between two and four times in our lives?

By expanding our vision to place ourselves within the wider cosmos as well as focusing our vision to center our humanity within our heart, we can begin to understand more about what makes up a human being and our place within the wider world. We can begin to understand how and why things deteriorate, suffer, grow ill—and how to bring about healing.

For the record, I am not actually suggesting that we some-how convince ourselves that the sun revolves around the Earth. That perspective belongs to an earlier time. I'm suggesting that if we acknowledge the connections between human beings, the heart, and the wider cosmos that have been lost or severed and work to heal them, perhaps we can arrive at a new—even more enlightened—place of love, trust, security, and health.

CHAPTER ELEVEN

A Heart of Gold

It's well known that one of the biggest risk factors for poor health is poverty.[1] Countless studies have examined the relationship between obesity and poverty;[2] between diabetes and poverty;[3] between mental illness and poverty;[4] between heart disease and poverty.[5]

As with the term *heart disease*, it's important, if challenging, to define and contextualize what we're talking about when we refer to poverty. Simplistically put, poverty can be defined as "the state of one who lacks a usual or socially acceptable amount of money or material possessions."[6] And there are various benchmarks to define this in the United States and worldwide. For example, in one report issued by the Pew Research Center, anyone living on less than two dollars a day is considered poor.[7] In 2016, the US federal poverty line was $11,880 for a household of one and $24,300 for a family of four.[8] But what does it mean to live on $2 a day in Swaziland versus $2 a day in India? Or $11,880 in rural Kentucky versus $11,800 in San Francisco?

More importantly, is money the only measure of what it means to suffer from poverty? And if there is such a strong correlation between poverty and poor health, will it ever really be possible to improve people's health without taking on industrial capitalism, income inequality, and injustice of every stripe? It seems significant that while poverty has supposedly declined in the United States and worldwide in recent years, the rate of chronic disease has climbed and is expected to continue to do so.[9]

In 1939, Weston A. Price published his landmark book, *Nutrition and Physical Degeneration*, following extensive ethnographic nutritional studies of communities and cultures around the world including Polynesians, Native Americans, Aborigines, and the Lötschental in Switzerland. It was a significant moment in history to study the intersection between nutrition and traditional communities since both were undergoing rapid and monumental changes. The moment provided Dr. Price with an opportunity to observe communities whose nutritional (and other) habits had changed significantly and those that hadn't— or hadn't yet.

Dr. Price found that where a diet high in sugar and processed foods had not taken hold, inhabitants were models of long, disease-free living—even though many had no money at all. They were neither living in poverty, nor did they have poor health. This suggests that the real risk factor for poor health and disease is having less money than those around you in societies where one needs money to procure the basic necessities of life and to avoid living in conditions that are rife with social and physical toxins. Certainly, this appears to be true in the United States today.

However, research is also emerging that suggests we still have a ways to go before we will fully understand the relationship between poverty and disease.[10] To me, that means we also still have a ways to go before we can say that raising the standard of living worldwide—as defined by employment, wealth, comfort, and possession of material goods—via our present path of growth-driven industrial capitalism is the quickest route to a greater well-being for all. I don't think that, as a society, we'll ever be able to buy our way to good health even though this may be possible in some individual cases.

———◆———

Since our relationship to money is so intimately connected to our health, I've always been interested in what money is, how it is controlled, and how it relates to the heart in particular. Our relationship to gold, especially, fascinates me. Gold (element 79, or Au) has, for millennia, been used as money and a symbol of power. This connection between gold and money persisted since well before Roman times until 1973 when Richard Nixon shocked the world and took the United States off the gold standard (although to some extent, it still remains). This marked the first time in American history that wealth had no official connection to gold and could not be redeemed for it. Most people would explain this long-standing connection between wealth and gold as having arisen because gold is relatively rare, immutable (it doesn't deteriorate over time), and can be easily divided into any size you wish. Fair enough, but I am convinced that there is more to it than that.

Pharaohs and kings have traditionally used gold to demonstrate their power and connection to the divine. Gold crowns have been the jewelry of choice, possibly because the crown of our heads also suggests a connection with authority and higher worlds. The story of gold shows up in places like the Old Testament, where Moses chides the people for worshipping the golden calf on their way out of Egypt and slavery. And it appears in fairy tales such as "Rapunzel," suggesting a mysticism underlying the metal. Yet the reality is that besides being shiny and resistant to most Earth forces (think rust), there is not much you can do with gold. So what's the big deal with gold? And what is money anyway?

As I mentioned in chapter 1, as a child, I often struggled to understand why things were the way they were in the adult world. Adult explanations often made no sense to me at all. Growing up near Detroit and being exposed to its urban decay at a young age, I couldn't help but wonder why there were so many destroyed neighborhoods and boarded-up houses and why there was so much trash everywhere. The decayed houses were real, the people living in poverty were real, the materials needed to refurbish these houses existed in abundance, and there were thousands of people in Detroit who had no jobs and might love the opportunity to rebuild their houses and those of their neighbors. It wasn't the case that there weren't enough skilled people to provide training to rebuild homes and communities. These people also existed in abundance. So why do neighborhoods in Detroit, St. Louis, Iraq, Palestine, and thousands of other places across the world continue to decay?

Likewise, we have forests that have been clear-cut, toxic dumpsites that need to be remediated, rivers that need to be un-dammed, mountains that have had their tops removed with wastelands left in their place. These things are *real*. These problems are real and need to be addressed to restore our world to health and wholeness. And, again, the knowledge exists. People who have no jobs—or meaningless jobs—exist in abundance. The materials needed to do these jobs already exist, so no new "resources" need be used to carry out these tasks. So, why on Earth does nothing get done? Why do we tolerate the crying needs of people, plants, animals, and the Earth for something to be done? Why do these cries fall on deaf ears?

To an adult, the answer is simple. There is no money.

But unlike all of these people and needs, which are real, money does not actually exist. It is only make-believe. The reason we tolerate all this misery and decay is *make-believe*, no more grounded in reality than wishing the Easter bunny would come hopping along to solve these problems for us. Aren't children supposed to live in a world of make-believe? Or is it the adults who do?

Imagine a world in which money is needed to obtain goods and services in order to live. This should not be hard because it's the world we already live in. So imagine both you and I want to buy a house for our families. We have similar-sized families, and we both want to buy the same house. The owner puts his house up for sale, and we both submit offers. In this imaginary scenario, instead of our current monetary system based on dollars (and loosely on gold), the money is called Cowans and I, Tom Cowan, am the only one who is allowed to make Cowans. I can make as many Cowans as I want, and everyone else has to work to obtain my Cowans in order to make any purchases or the Cowan police will put them in jail. If your society rebels against this arrangement, the Cowan military will change the regime in your country. When we go to bid on the house, I will always win. I will continue to win until I own everything and the rest of the people will have nothing. There will, of course, be friends and family members whom I shower with Cowans. Occasionally I allow a chosen few to also make a lot of Cowans under certain conditions, but eventually "my people" and I will own it all. In fact, the only real constraint on my owning everything is that there will be so few Cowan insiders compared to everyone else, that if I get overzealous in acquiring everything, people might get upset and either stop making things I want or, heaven forbid, string me up by my neck. So, I must be careful and possibly even not let on that this is how the whole situation works.

Sounds bizarre, right? But this is how our financial system works. Just change the name from Cowans to dollars and Cowan friends and families to international banking friends and families and read this paragraph again.

How can this be? How, as adults, can we tolerate this?

We live in a situation in which we have been fooled into thinking our money is made by the government—in other words, us—when in reality, most money is created out of thin air by a privately held bank called the Federal Reserve and the other chartered banks that rule international finance.[11] This money they create is attached now to nothing, not even to gold. It is not connected to deposits made by depositors, not to assets, not to skill in money management. When you go to the bank for a loan or mortgage, they create the money they loan you. Then they add interest to ensure that there will never be enough money in the system to handle all the need. This is done by a stroke of the keyboard on the computer. The amazing part of this system of money creation is that most people accept it and some will give their lives to make sure it can continue. Money created in this way is completely imaginary. It is based on nothing in the "real" world. As with my above example, eventually the bankers will own everything, with the caveat that if they get too aggressive, the hoi polloi might rebel.

The Bretton Woods Agreement of the 1940s established that most international trade, especially the crucial oil we use to power our economies, must be conducted in dollars. Since the United States is the only country that can create dollars, the rest of the world has to "work" to obtain our dollars. We will eventually make nothing and do nothing, and our culture will be devoted to money management. (Typically this is referred to in more dignified terms: We will be economists and financial planners.) If another country decides the system is rigged against them and tries to sell their wares in currency other than dollars, they will be targeted for regime change (a euphemism for taking a functional society—one that, while loaded with problems, has water, food, and housing for its people—and reducing it to rubble). When Saddam Hussein tried to sell oil in currencies besides dollars, it was time for regime change.[12] When Qaddafi tried to start a pan-African currency to compete with the dollar, it was time for regime change.[13] Iran, Russia, Syria, and perhaps China are next, subject to whether they decide to fall in line behind the dollar and the extent to which the population—both theirs and ours—can be manipulated or coerced. Don't misunderstand me. This is not a vote of support or an excuse for the practices of these dictators or these countries. It's quite likely that, given the chance, they would likewise force the world to trade in rubles—or whatever other kind of fantasy money they can cook up.

So there is this aspect of gold that we associate with money, in all its bizarre manifestations. How is it that something real— gold—can stand for something invented? If we allow our imaginations to work in this way, perhaps we could allow our imaginations to entertain the idea of something that seems invented or magical—or just a little too out there for our mechanistically trained brains to be comfortable with—and consider whether it might be something real. It's this aspect of gold—I think of it as gold's cosmic side—that intrigues me most. It makes me wonder whether it might offer a path out of our current global catastrophe and what it might teach us about healing the heart. Bear with me as we travel down the road of modern-day alchemy.

There is no significant amount of gold, as we know it, to be found in our heart or in our circulation. Gold is found as a trace element in our blood, but no one to my knowledge has claimed that it has any particular physiological or pathological significance. Like silver, gold is a noble metal, all of which resist corrosion and oxidation and, according to most people, are incapable of the lack of electrical resistance that characterizes superconductivity. However, some people argue—and this is, admittedly, on the fringes of accepted science—that there is a "pure" form of gold that is as significant to humanity as the alchemists who sought it for centuries believed it was.

This form of gold is known as Orbitally Rearranged Monoatomic Elements (ORME, or ORMUS)—a cumbersome name for a phenomenon that is anything but. ORME describes a change in form that can occur in gold, silver, and the platinum metals. In gold as we know it—earthly, rather than cosmic, gold, so to speak—electrons circle the nucleus and are available to form bonds with other atoms, resulting in compounds such as gold chloride. Under certain vortex-creating conditions, however, the atoms can pull in their electrons and assume a high-speed condensed form. In this form, it's impossible to connect with other elements to form compounds. Like a figure skater who pulls her arms in to spin faster, the electrons are pulled in toward the nucleus as the atoms spin faster and faster. Elements in this state are referred to as monoatomic, although they can form in pairs or even triplets, and they are called elemental because they can no longer form connections with other elements.

ORME exhibit some amazing properties. For example, they can no longer conduct heat or electricity; typically silver and gold compound wires are among the best conductors of heat and electricity. They also, inexplicably, have a different weight—always lighter than their conventional counterparts, subjected less to gravity than to levity. And while ORME elements can't conduct heat or electricity, they become superconductors of sorts, capable of conducting a variety of "impulses" virtually at the speed of light. This dramatically reduces the friction, and hence the energy required, and dramatically increases the speed at which something can travel. Lastly, and probably most eyebrow raising, is that ORME elements cannot be measured by conventional atomic measuring devices such as spectrophotometers because these devices depend on the interaction of the element and the device. ORME elements don't interact with other elements, nor with measuring devices, so they can't be detected. With this in mind, allow me a couple of digressions.

If you ask a physiologist or a neurologist how a nerve works, they will likely respond with some variation of the following answer. Nerves are made up of a bundle of nerve cells (neurons) that transmit information through electrical and chemical signals via long, slender (and hydrophilic, by the way) projections known as axons that terminate in synapses. These electrochemical nerve impulses are carried unidirectionally inside these axons, which are insulated with a fatty coating called myelin, like copper wires insulated by rubber casings, and they arise from gradients in ions such as calcium and magnesium. The nerve impulse is carried along the length of the nerve by the movement of these ions until a neurotransmitter—for example, serotonin, dopamine, or acetylcholine—is released from the presynaptic junction. This neurotransmitter essentially swims across the junction and attaches to a receptor site on the postsynaptic junction, where it causes a depolarization of the next neuron. The next impulse travels unidirectionally down this nerve to the next synapse and so on. The nerve eventually ends at its destination, such as a muscle, which it "fires," resulting in planned action, such as movement.

This sequence seems clear and well worked out. In medicine, we routinely manipulate neurotransmitters to affect disease processes—such as serotonin in depression and dopamine in Parkinson's. And we know that if the myelin is damaged, it will disturb impulse transmission and therefore neurological dysfunction. This is considered to be the underlying pathophysiology of such illnesses as multiple sclerosis (MS), amyotrophic lateral sclerosis (ALS), and other "de-myelinating" diseases. All very clear and precise, right?

Now do the following. It's best to have a partner to help you. Put both index fingers out in front of you. Then close your eyes and have your partner say either right or left. (You can do it yourself if you have to, but the results are not as convincing.) As soon as your partner says right or left, wiggle that index finger. Do it three times. Now answer this question. How long did it take between hearing the word "right" or "left" and wiggling your index finger? I have done this with thousands of people, and most people say, "Only a few seconds."

"You mean I say 'right' and then 'one one thousand,' 'two one thousand,' and then you wiggle your finger?" I ask.

"No, much shorter," they reply.

"How much shorter?"

Most people I can bargain down to about 1/100th of a second, but really it's virtually instantaneous.

Now comes the crucial question: Do you believe that the time it takes for the sound wave from my voice to wiggle your ear drum, then stimulate the acoustic nerve, which then conducts this impulse sequentially along the nerve via a changing gradient of calcium and magnesium ions before the impulse ends at a "moat," releasing a neurotransmitter, which then swims across the moat—it helps to dramatize this with a swimming motion at this point—until it finds its appropriate mooring and sets off the next chemical depolarization is 1/100th of a second, or virtually instantaneous? Probably not, and you haven't even wiggled your finger yet!

After ten to twenty of these nerve transmissions, the impulse arrives at the brain. Inside the brain, it circles around for a while and then exits out the motor neurons. Finally it arrives at your finger, stimulating the coordinated motion of dozens of muscles inside your finger. And yet our experience of this is that it happens instantaneously. For me, I can't believe that this is accurate. The process is too fast and too coordinated. There must something else at work that has nothing to do with neurotransmitters, synapses, or the flow of calcium within the nerve cells.

This is the reason I talked about the sun going around the Earth in chapter 10. Our direct experience screams out to us, "This is what I see. This is what I experience." Then science, or industrial capitalism, or "adulthood," comes along and serves up an explanation that, while sort of true, just doesn't make sense. Scientific explanations often take us further from that crucial place of trust in ourselves. The task of the modern human is to reconcile both the place of trust in oneself and the role (and, at times, usefulness) of these scientific explanations. No scientific explanation can really explain to me how a nerve works. The process is just too fast, too instantaneous. Maybe, better put, it exists almost out of time. The old Newtonian billiard ball explanation of reality is simply not adequate to explain what I, for one, experience of life.

To borrow a concept from physics, we seem to be quantum coherent organisms, the basis of which is the instantaneous flow of electrons—like electricity or wireless technology that seems to act out of the normal flow of time—over space. So the sound impulse from my voice creates phenomena throughout the body almost instantaneously. Without this ability to coordinate muscle activity instantaneously, life would not be possible. The chemical effects that neurologists, doctors, and physiologists focus on are the *results* of this quantum superconduction. It's no wonder we can't successfully treat so many neurological diseases. We don't actually have a clue about how a nerve works. We are mostly just busy studying and manipulating the effects of the phenomena.

Now imagine the following story: There is a famous animal tracker who long ago went into the woods to track animals. All was as usual until he ran across a track he had never seen before. It was in the shape of a two-dimensional chestahedron. He was perplexed because he had never encountered an animal whose hooves could have made this impression. But they were clearly animal tracks, and he also found some scat nearby. He named the animal Lynda after his beloved wife. He set about looking for this new Lynda animal, seeing more and more tracks but never actually finding this shy, elusive animal. He showed other trackers the tracks. They all agreed that these tracks could only have been made by a hitherto unknown animal, but nobody was ever successful in finding the Lynda.

Eventually the original tracker died, but the mystery of the tracks remained. This became a subject of great scientific interest.

As the decades and centuries went by with still no sighting of the animal, many theories began to emerge. Most claimed that, in fact, these tracks were not made by a mythical animal at all but were the result of substances in the soil. Scientists studied which elements were present in the clearest footprints. They studied how much water was needed in the soil to make the best prints. And so on. Chairs in major universities were created for those who had the best understanding of the conditions in the soil and atmosphere that would create the best and clearest tracks. Even Nobel Prizes were awarded to those with the clearest theories as to how the earth's elements give rise to the tracks. Alternative theories based on astrological events and grand conspiracies were also proposed to explain the mysterious tracks.

Then one day a little girl who loved all sorts of animals went walking in the woods. The woods contained many of these chestahedron tracks, and the little girl came across a small deer-like animal that had fallen and hurt her legs. She carefully carried the animal back home to her parents to see if someone could help the poor, lame animal. The townspeople were amazed. The small animal, very shy of course, had chestahedron-shaped hooves. The mystery was finally solved. This was the long sought after animal who had, all this time, been making the tracks.

The little girl and her family nursed the animal back to health, and then, with great excitement, they brought the animal to the great university to show the professors. "Look, the mystery is solved," the little girl exclaimed. But the professors were skeptical. They had the Lynda tested to see if it could be true that this animal, not the forces of the earth, had been making the tracks all this time. They had the Lynda walk on concrete—no tracks. On a gymnasium floor—no tracks. In water—still no tracks. They concluded that the Lynda, even though it had some interesting features—that is, hooves shaped like the chestahedron tracks—could not possibly be responsible for the tracks. They concluded, as they had said all along, that the earth was responsible for the tracks.

The Lynda was making the tracks all along. She was just hard to find, shy as she is. It was also true, however, that without the earth, the Lynda could leave no tracks and that, as the scientists claimed, different compositions of minerals, soils, and water affected the quality and even presence of the tracks. I believe it is the same with our nerves and, in fact, with everything in living systems. In nerves, it is the superconducted quantum coherence that is the true nerve impulse. This organizes the body into a coherent organism. And it leaves behind a chemical footprint as it passes through the nerves.

As in our story, without the chemicals, no nervous activity is possible. And, as in our story, the integrity of the chemicals affects the transmission, or footprints. But they are not, and never could be, the cause. It is this confusion between footprint and cause that leaves conventional medicine so powerless to identify the root of most illnesses and equally powerless to cure them. I am not suggesting that changing the effects won't affect an outcome. It can, sometimes even in very positive ways. But it can't find or treat the cause.

So how then does this quantum cohesion phenomenon occur in the nerves? First of all, axons are hydrophilic "tubes" well suited to structuring the water inside our nerve cells. Structured water, as we know, creates an electrical charge that results in movement. And we know that electricity can carry impulses almost instantaneously even over tremendous distances. As with circulation, the structured water and the flow of electrons is the force behind the nerve transmission, leaving a chemical footprint in its wake.

But living beings seem like more than electrical impulse devices. Even that seems too slow, too simplistic, too reductionist. I believe that what we call *life*—and what Steiner called the etheric body—is the transformation of a chemically based "substance" to a quantum coherent superconducting phenomenon. Life is, always, more than the sum of its parts. And life is not life when it is reduced to those parts. I believe that the reason we are struggling to treat human illnesses—and to effectively care for our ecosystems and communities—is that we do not even have the proper foundation to distinguish life from non-life. Absent a coherent conception of life, doctors are forced to treat life as if it obeyed the laws of non-living, material substances. But I don't think it does. I think we are coherent, electrically charged, superconducting, light-filled beings, and this foundation needs to be the basis of medicine—as well as of a healing process for all life on earth. *Disease, health, life*—these are verbs, not nouns. They are dynamic processes, a constant flux and flow and interchange, and I don't know how we can ever effectively treat people until we begin to see things this way.

Where does the superconducting "material" come from? Indulge me in some speculation: Gold is the most prominent and important orbitally rearranged monoatomic element and was perhaps, after all, what sages, alchemists, and spiritual seekers all over the world have been after for millennia. It is the ORME, or cosmic form of gold, that is the primary superconducting matrix without which nerve transmission and life itself would not be possible.

The most effective way to transform earthly gold into cosmic gold is to put it into a high-speed vortex device. The faster a vortex spins, the colder the center becomes, defying the way substances usually behave because typically the faster something moves, the warmer it becomes. This high-speed vortex is created by the chestahedron shape of the heart as described by Frank Chester. Is it possible, then, that the heart of gold refers to its unique ability to carry out this transformation of an earthly element into cosmic gold, thereby providing the basis for life to exist?

I realize that this may seem like a stretch, but think back to the invention of money. Ask yourself whether you know that the earth revolves around the sun and, if so, how you *know* that the earth revolves around the sun. Is it because you have observed retrograde movement of the planets, or is it because you have been told it and because it would be ridiculous to believe otherwise? What do you know, in your heart, to be true? In the next chapter, I will explore the final stage of our heart-centered journey, which is what we mean by love, possibly one of the few things most of us do know to be true. And where does that knowledge come from, if not from our heart?

CHAPTER TWELVE

What's Love Got to Do with It?

D r. Paul Pearsall was a neuropsychologist who counseled patients before and after they underwent heart transplant surgery. In his 1999 book, *The Heart's Code*, Dr. Pearsall described the profound effects a new heart can have on a transplant recipient. He found that many of the heart transplant patients he worked with experienced a significant and inexplicable change in their personality—or, as I think of it, the essence of their being—following the receipt of a new heart. Shockingly, this new essence often reflected the essence of the organ donor.

There could be many explanations for this change of heart, so to speak. Receiving a heart transplant is a terrifying and traumatic experience that forces people to confront their own mortality in a direct, even brutal, way. And patients are given powerful medications before, during, and after surgery, including medications to prevent their bodies from rejecting a new organ; these drugs can have short- and long-term psychological effects. Patients may also experience profound relief after they receive a new, healthier heart—the heady and overwhelming feeling of having a new lease on life that can alter someone's entire perspective on life. Profound emotional and psychological upheaval in a patient could be considered a very normal and healthy reaction to the intensity of undergoing and surviving a heart transplant operation.

But this can't fully explain what Dr. Pearsall heard from his patients. In *The Heart's Code*, he tells the story of a white, middle-aged man who worked all his life in a factory, espoused racist beliefs, and had no interest in what some might refer to as high-brow culture such as opera and classical music. Then this man received a new heart from an anonymous donor. In the weeks and months that followed, as the man recovered, his wife began to witness profound changes in him—describing a husband who seemed almost like a new man. He wasn't simply relieved and grateful and shaken by the experience of having undergone a heart transplant. He started to hang out in places that were mostly frequented by African Americans. He became friends with African American coworkers whom he had previously shunned and found no common ground with. He even seemed to walk differently. And eventually, mostly in secret, he began to listen to classical music, especially violin concertos.

For months, this man attempted to hide these personality changes, conflicted between the man he had been and the man he had become. Inevitably, the change of heart prevailed and he was able to embrace a new life, a new essence. Deeply curious, the man and his wife began to investigate the identity of the donor. They discovered that he was a young African American male who had been shot and killed while walking to school. This was mysterious and fascinating to them, but their profound awe came years later when they learned further details—that the young man was shot and killed on his way to the music academy at which he was studying to be a classical violinist.

There are many other stories like this. And because organ donations often come from people who are otherwise healthy and suffer a violent death, there have also been cases in which a heart recipient has been able to help the police solve a crime based on their intimate knowledge of how events unfolded on the day "they" died. The recipient, of course, wasn't there, had never met or heard of the previous heart's "owner," and had no "earthly" way of knowing how events transpired. But he or she is—somehow—able to provide accurate and verifiable details as leads for the investigators.[1]

In *The Heart's Code*, Dr. Pearsall explains that his approach in helping transplant patients adjust to their new heart is to try to help them stop listening to their conscious, logical reasons and to try to just "flow" with their actual, present experience. Most of us have had this experience and know the difference between the state of consciousness when your mind is constantly going, analyzing, thinking, worrying, planning and those profound, if rare, moments when you are in the moment, just being, when the relentless machinations of your mind seem to have fallen away.

Dr. Pearsall describes some transplant recipients who are never able to achieve this in a meaningful way. They seem to have no new memories or "essence." Often these patients never stop struggling to cope with their posttransplant reality. The patients who either naturally or, through Dr. Pearsall's counseling accept or even embrace new memories and a new essence often have the best health outcomes. At that point, many even revel in their change of heart—and their whole new life.

These changes have not been observed in patients with kidney, liver, or lung transplants. It seems that only with a new heart do you get a new "personality." And this new personality comes with a choice, the freedom to choose between suppressing or embracing it. Some people suppress it, and often the rest of their lives are full of tremendous struggle and conflict. Others choose to accept this change of heart, flow with it, eager—if fearful—to see where it takes them. Although this phenomenon is most dramatic among heart transplant recipients, who among us has not had an experience like this? Standing at a crossroads, often after a tragic, traumatic, or terrifying experience such as a chronic illness or accident, you are faced with the choice between desperately trying to hang on to life as you knew it—a life that, while familiar and therefore comfortable, may no longer be right for you—and a frightening but exhilarating leap of faith where you are guided only by something powerful inside of you, something that seems to reside in your heart and that gives you the courage to move forward in an unknown direction without fear.

When I met my wife Lynda, it was like getting a new heart. She was a gift from somewhere I didn't know existed and couldn't really understand. But I had a choice to make, too. I could reorient my life around this new reality or choose to not be bothered because the new way had so many uncertainties and so much uncharted territory ahead. I believe it is love that gives us the courage to make this choice, this leap of faith. And where we find love, we inexorably find the heart. It is the core of our being, the keeper of our essence.

What does the heart have to do with love? Probably nothing, according to your cardiologist. The heart is a finely innervated piece of specialized muscle. Nothing else exists but this physical stuff. Dissection of the heart reveals nothing one can call love. The heliocentric, modern, scientific, quantitative, double-blind research, mechanistic paradigm says there is no connection between the heart and love. And yet, across centuries and across cultures, so many countless people—poets, writers, lovers, mothers, fathers, children, even scientists—have experienced love and have connected it with the heart. What gives? Where lies the truth?

I can't define love or characterize it in a succinct way. But I do know that love, perhaps more than any other feeling, involves our essential self. You do not love something in a superficial way. Superficiality and love are mutually exclusive.

But what is meant by our essential self? Imagine yourself as a young child playing in a park. Then picture yourself as a teenager, as a young adult, and then as a middle-aged or elderly person walking with a slower, stiffer gait. It doesn't matter whether you've reached old age yet or not. Physically, the cells in your body—those things that scientists and doctors "believe" in—are different in each of those scenarios because your body replaces your cells over time. Nothing is the same between that young child playing in the park and that elder walking slowly and gingerly.

And yet we all know there is a thread, an essence, that runs through each of our lives. We know there is continuity between the child who was and the elder who will be. Although it's impossible to articulate a person's essence without it sounding glib, I believe Mozart's essence—and the reason he was able to give us so much—had something to do with the tension between his musical genius and his immaturity. Tiger Woods's essence has something to do with an almost mystical connection to golf and the natural consequences of a lost childhood. Dostoyevsky's essence had to do with justice and freedom; these ideas, those deeply held beliefs permeated everything he wrote and did throughout his life. For me, my essence has to do with trying to get to the heart of a matter, of a deep unease with answers that are served on a platter, an essence that has kept me company through my entire life. This essence seems to arrive at or before birth and travel with us at least until the day we die.

This essence is also revealed in the way we refer to ourselves spatially. If you want to make a gesture referring to yourself, you don't point to your foot and say, "This is me." You don't point to your genitals, or abdomen, or buttocks, or even your head and say, "This is me." Try it. It feels weird and wrong. Then point to your heart and see if you feel, "There do I dwell."

Scientific, maybe not. An actual experience, absolutely. And again there is the question of which do you trust as a way of knowing? When you want to connect with another person, do you hold them to your foot, your buttocks, or against your head? (Try this with a child or a beloved pet. I strongly suspect it will feel weird and wrong.) No, you hold your beloved against your heart. We have an instinct to represent deep connection with our heart—far and above the fact that it is convenient for our arms to reach that part of anatomy. Even cardiologists don't hold their children against their buttocks when their children feel sad or hurt.

If we want to convey a deeply held belief, we often hold our clenched fist—about the same size and shape as our heart—over our hearts. We don't hold it over our head or over our abdomen. (Again, try it and see how it feels.) When we want to make an emotional connection, convey our deep feelings, or demonstrate that we are dealing with our "essence" as a human, we rush to get our heart involved in the experience.

Love necessarily involves the deepest part of our being, our essence. Nobody, not even the most cynical among us, wants to be told, "I love you with all my foot," or "My brain loves you very much," or, even worse, "My genitals are in love with you." No one wants to hear that. We only accept expressions of the heart as meaningful.

Like essence, freedom is also necessarily part of the definition of love. For it to be love, a person needs to tell you—and, more importantly, show you through freely chosen actions—that being with you, fighting for you, protecting you, caring for you is a path they have freely chosen. There is no such thing as loving you because I had no choice, loving you because there was a gun to my head, loving you to impress my dad, or loving you because economically it was the soundest choice. This kind of "love" either doesn't last or becomes the worst kind of torture. For love, there must be choice. But perhaps more precisely, there must be choice within the inexorability of the connection. It is as if the world somehow presents you with the possibility, but you are then compelled to follow the path—as if something powerful inside guides you along it, whatever your brain may say.

Afterword

There are many ways to conceive of a life. I like to conceive of life as a musical score. You sound a central theme in the opening of the piece, play on this theme a bit, and then proceed to explore as many ideas as possible in that key. As the piece progresses, you delve deeper and deeper into the central theme with growing clarity, sophistication, and audacity. All the while, you continue to explore related ideas without ever losing the connection or straying too far from your central theme. When you approach the finale, if all has gone well, you come to some resolution of the idea of the piece. If you are lucky, you find a sort of peace or harmony, or maybe acceptance, of the themes you have grappled with throughout your life.

Although I hope I'm not too close to the finale yet, this book has been that resolution for me—and understanding the heart its central theme. While I certainly hope to learn and understand more about the heart as I step into my sixth decade, it felt like time to take stock of where I have come thus far. Meeting my grandchildren—Ben, Sam, and Amiya—catalyzed that feeling in me.

Ben is our first grandchild, the first child of my daughter, Molly, and son-in-law, Andrew. Lynda met Ben before I did, having traveled to New Hampshire to help Molly move while Ben was still an infant. Lynda returned home intrigued with Ben, remarking that she would often look over at Ben only to see him smiling at her as if to get her attention or interact with her in some way. When I met Ben, it was love at first sight. I learned what a world of difference there is between being a parent and being a grandparent. Being a grandparent comes with no expectations and fewer anxieties. You don't worry about whether they behave right or meet their milestones. It's more like meeting pure joy.

When Ben was two and a half years old, Molly and the two boys spent a month with us in San Francisco while Andrew was away for work. When I returned home from work, Ben would jump up from his blocks as soon as he heard the door open, and I would hear, "Gampa's home!" He would run into my arms, and we would smile and hug. Then he would take me by the hand to show me his farm. I would give him his "present" from the day, usually a tongue depressor. (Wow, a new sword!) We would work together on the farm he was building out of blocks, go water the "real" garden, pick our dinner's vegetables, and sometimes feed the chickens and worms.

Just living—the flow of gifts from one to the other. I cried a lot when it was time for Ben and Sam to go home. Grandparenting may be the final, best gift we ever receive in our lives. It reconnects us to life in a way that has largely faded away with the joy and excitement of childhood. Of course, the grandchildren will grow up and maybe start to wonder about this old guy, as they naturally grow more and more interested in their independent lives. But for now, as I live in the flow of this incredible gift—hang out with Lynda, tend my garden, ask my patients about their lives, and build farms out of blocks with my grandchildren—I can't help but take stock. And, while I hate to give recipes, here is what I know about caring for the heart:

- Eat good food and only good food. Start with *Nourishing Traditions* and adjust from there.
- Drink only good water—water that is pure, mineralized, and structured. Visit www.dancingwithwater.com and explore from there.
- Get as much sun exposure (without burning) as you can.
- Walk with your bare feet on the earth as much as possible, especially at beaches, lakes, rivers, and oceans. Play—with bare feet—in the water.
- Try to restore to health as many living beings as you can. This can include plants, animals, mountains, fields, rivers, lakes, relationships, and other people. Everything around us is alive. Find the living beings you care about, nurture them, be the one responsible for ensuring their well-being. Love them, protect them, fight for them, care for them.

Finally, maybe most importantly, shed as many of your beliefs as possible, including those so-called cherished ones. Be wary of believing in any institutions or abstractions (i.e., nations, patriotism, capitalism). Ask yourself what you know to be true in your heart versus what you've been told. Only knowing comes from your heart. When you have done enough of this shedding that it has become a habit, turn around in line every once in a while and see who and what is there. If who or what is there moves your heart (you'll know), stop at nothing to make this who or what a part of your life.

The Cowan Heart Diet

Any rational therapy must proceed from a thorough understanding of the cause of what you wish to treat. With heart disease, the most important underlying issue that we can influence with diet is the inflammation of the blood vessels. Current theory as to the reason for the plaque buildup in the blood vessels is that the plaque is a therapeutic response to chronic inflammation in the arteries. This inflammatory response is one of the manifestations of the metabolic syndrome that was discussed in chapter 7. The diet therapy is a key component in reversing the metabolic syndrome. Rather than give you a list of foods to eat or not eat, this dietary advice will give you sound principles that will allow you to construct a diet that works for you and will help you achieve better metabolic health. I've included a few sample menus at the end to give you an idea of how to apply these principles. There are six principles of the Cowan Heart Diet:

Principle One: Quality Matters

The first principle of the Cowan Heart Diet is that this is a quality-based diet. This means that all the food you eat must be the best quality available to you and, in some cases, that you can afford. The principle that guides me in assessing food quality is simple: It should be grown in a manner that is the healthiest for the living being that we are about to eat. This means that the healthiest chicken to eat is a chicken grown in a way that is best for that chicken. We can never achieve health by eating sick plants or animals. This makes for reasonably straightforward decision making. We start with asking a simple question: Under what conditions would that carrot, chicken, or salmon thrive? Here are some rules of thumb:

1. Animal foods. When choosing foods from animals, land, or sea, choose the animals grown in a way that is most compatible with the nature of that animal. Cows are healthiest when kept on pasture. Fish are healthiest when allowed to forage freely in oceans, lakes, or rivers. Chickens need to scratch and forage in the fields, and pigs need time to dig in the forest with their snouts. By allowing the animals to freely express their unique nature, we are not only honoring the sacrifices of these animals but also ensuring that we are eating healthy animals, as well as contributing to a functioning ecosystem.

2. Seed food. This category includes seeds, nuts, grains, and legumes. While I can in no way pretend to understand the likes and dislikes of an almond tree, I can imagine that all plants "enjoy" growing in a diverse ecosystem rather than in the mono-crop environment of conventional agriculture. One of the best biodynamic gardeners I know always plants one or two herbs or flowers in every vegetable bed to "give the vegetables something beautiful to look at." Some people will say this is crazy because vegetables don't have eyes, but

we know that biodiversity is related to resilience and that growing many different plants together is one of the best ways to ward off pests and ensure the health of our food plants. The permaculture food forest concept teaches that growing nut trees alongside other food crops, often as a kind of understory, improves the health of the soil and the health of the trees, and can also maximize yields. For these reasons, seed food should be grown in diverse, organic, biodynamic, or permaculture environments whenever possible.

In terms of preparation, seed foods should be soaked for twelve to twenty-four hours or sprouted before cooking. This simple step breaks down some of the antinutrients contained in the seed that keep the seed dormant. Soaking or sprouting seeds, nuts, grains, and legumes makes them easier to cook, taste better, and more digestible.

3. Vegetables and fruit. In general, the percentage of vegetable to fruit consumption should be about 80 percent vegetable, 20 percent fruit. Again, these foods should all be sustainably grown. This is covered in greater detail in Principle Two.

Principle Two: How to Eat Vegetables

Drawing on the documented diets of healthy traditional peoples, my experience living in rural Swaziland for two years, and USDA guidelines, I have reached the conclusion that even the most health conscious Americans live in a veritable food desert when it comes to vegetable intake. Traditional peoples often ate a huge number of and variety of vegetables. This diversity included many root vegetables, many different types of leaves, and many "fruit" vegetables, such as squash. Members of the Miwok tribe in Northern California consumed about 120 different kinds of vegetables per year. Some of these were perennials, some were annuals, some were planted in gardens, and others were gathered from the fields and forests. There is evidence that they tended the entirety of the land on which they dwelled to ensure an adequate supply of vegetables in their diets, as well as to ensure sufficient habitat for the animals that they hunted.

People in some parts of the United States have access to healthy sources of the animal products, grains, seeds, nuts, and beans I recommend. However, even in the food-rich Bay Area where I live, very few people have access to 120 different kinds of vegetables. In particular, almost everyone lacks adequate amounts of perennial vegetables, which, due to their extensive root systems are able to "mine" the soil for nutrients that are often unavailable to annual plants.

Perennial plants also often develop a more robust defense system than their annual relatives. This means they produce an abundance of protective chemicals that are meant to protect the plant against disease and predation. These same defenses also help animals who eat them to ward off diseases. For example, Ashitaba (in the *Angelica* genus) contains the cancer-fighting chemical chalcones in its stem. You don't need to be a botanist or biochemist to eat a healthy diet. But you do need to understand the principles of a diverse vegetable diet. This means eating small amounts of at least five to ten different vegetables per day. You should eat green vegetables (leaves), red/orange vegetables (carrots/beets/squash), white vegetables (onions, leeks, garlic), and purple/black vegetables (tree collards, indigo apple tomatoes) on most days. You should include root vegetables, leaf vegetables, and fruit vegetables (squash, zucchini, peppers), as well as some annuals. See my booklet *How (and Why) to Eat More Vegetables* for more detailed guidelines.

Principle Three: Intermittent Fasting

Imagine you eat every eight hours of every day for your entire life. You eat right before bed and as soon as you wake up in the morning. Then you continue to eat at regular intervals throughout the day. What happens metabolically and hormonally to you?

For your entire life, you will be in a fed, or anabolic, state, meaning that you will be producing the hormones in your body, particularly insulin, that signal that you are "fed" and that any excess should be stored as fat. If this goes on, day after day, year after year, you will eventually get fatter and fatter, regardless of the content or quality of your food. The high insulin state would lead to a full-blown metabolic syndrome, which is the combination of obesity, high blood pressure (because insulin causes fluid retention, hence more pressure in the blood vessels), arthritis (insulin causes inflammation), diabetes, and other signs of degeneration. Nature has other plans for us, which is one reason we sleep and fast when we feel sick.

Our bodies are designed so that when we don't eat for twelve hours, we first run out of constituents in the food that keep our blood sugars within the normal range and then we run out of stored starch in our liver (glycogen), the next readily available source of blood sugar. Once this twelve-hour mark hits, our metabolic/hormonal state shifts, and we transition into a catabolic or breakdown phase. The main hormone of the catabolic state is glucagon, the antagonist of insulin. Glucagon catalyzes the mobilization, hence breakdown and turnover, of our fat stores in order to be the next line of defense against a dropping blood sugar. As this temporary fasting state continues, the body shifts more of the blood flow to our heart, brains, and muscles, possibly to get us more mentally and physically focused on finding some food. The hormone glucagon and the series of events that accompanies this catabolic state reduces inflammation wherever it may be occurring in the body. It also creates turnover of the fat cells so they can eliminate any stored toxins. The increased blood flow to the brain makes us more alert, focused, and sharp.

Anyone suffering from any type of imbalance related to deposition, such as plaque deposit in the arteries or calcium deposits in the joints, would be well served by regularly getting themselves into this temporary catabolic state. Nature and our bodies are so sophisticated that one explanation for getting sick is that we need to spend more time in this catabolic state; if we're not willing to do it consciously, through intermittent fasting, our inner wisdom will do it for us. We will get sick, stop eating, increase our temperature, flush out stored toxins, and then get back on our feet. Rather than living a life of chronic depositional disease or repeated acute illness, and the mental fogginess this goes along with, we can take matters into our hands through intermittent fasting.

Intermittent fasting is simple. It means going for twelve-plus hours without any food, especially any food or supplement that contains any trace of protein or carbohydrates. (Pure fats like coconut oil, ghee, and butter don't alter the hormonal events I described.) After twelve hours, you run out of glycogen and you start burning fat. If you extend this to seventeen or eighteen hours, one to six days per week, you have a powerful strategy to burn fat, lose weight, reverse diabetes, lower your blood pressure, reduce inflammation, and increase mental acuity. By many accounts, it is the single most effective antiaging strategy out there.[1]

To do this, eat an early dinner, finishing by 6 p.m. Go to bed and wake up at your normal time. Then instead of having your usual breakfast, drink plain water and do some vigorous activity (I like to garden if possible) until about noon. Eat your usual high-quality foods between noon and 6 p.m. Over time, you will feel the positive effects, and you will start to almost crave your fasting days for the sense of well-being they give you. It is one simple step that works for almost everyone in creating more robust health.

Principle Four:
Macronutrient Content of the Diet

Macronutrient composition refers to the three major components of our food: fats, proteins, and carbohydrates. Generally speaking, carbohydrates are used for energy production, proteins are used as the raw material for building the proteins and enzymes that are the structural and functional components of our bodies, and fats are used to regulate inflammation, make hormones, and as a secondary or backup fuel source. At least this is the scheme we are taught in biochemistry classes. It is becoming clear due to research into the ketogenic diet and neurological disease that fats are the best source of fuel for our hearts and brains, in particular.[2] These are also the two organs that consume the most fuel and oxygen in the human body.

Rudolf Steiner, in the only book he wrote about medicine, pointed out the crucial role of fat consumption in the prevention and treatment of degenerative disease. Steiner also suggested that fats from animals (i.e., butter) were the most efficient in creating the warmth humans need and use to prevent degeneration and aging. When speaking about warmth, we are in the realm of the heart because it is the heart that creates warmth, and it is the heart that preferentially uses fats as fuel. I do not recommend a low-fat diet for heart patients.

Grass-fed butter or ghee and the best quality coconut oil should be eaten with every meal and, if needed, as a fuel source between meals during fasting periods. Through the use of liberal fats combined with lowering of the carbohydrate intake, we eventually become fat adapted—a difficult term to define scientifically, but referring to the point at which a person can quickly convert ingested fats into an adequate amount of blood sugar. This adaptive ability varies greatly from person to person, so I don't offer patients fixed carbohydrate intake rules and limits. The idea is to create more flexibility in how you obtain energy from food.

Most Americans take the easy, harmful route of acquiring their energy from refined carbohydrates at regular intervals throughout the day, as opposed to high-quality fats and a small amount of the complex sugars from vegetables. You can assess how fat adapted you are if you stop all carbohydrate intake for a few days and see how you feel. Most people will feel listless, have low energy, and feel unwell because they're not able to run their metabolisms on fats for fuel.

The strategy I like to use is a gradual reduction of carbohydrates with a simultaneous gradual increase in grass-fed butter or ghee and coconut oil. As you wean yourself off refined and simple sugars, you add good fats slowly into your diet, and as you adjust to this, you also adjust the amount of starchy, allowed vegetables and fruit based on how you feel, especially with regards to your energy. If you are sluggish, eat more carbohydrate-rich fruits and vegetables. If your energy remains good, that means you are adapting to using the cleaner fats as fuel. Make these adjustments day to day, always attempting to eat only the amount of carbohydrates that your body seems to need. This diet is not a ketogenic diet, which, in my experience, is neither necessary nor advantageous. We need some carbohydrates in our diet, and we need the nutrients in the foods that contain carbohydrates. But we also need to develop flexibility in our metabolism—meaning the ability to convert fats into fuel. The strategy I outline here should allow you to gradually develop this flexibility.

Protein intake is another subject mired in controversy. My conclusion is that protein intake is vital, especially for the development of the many enzymes our bodies need, but that excessive protein intake isn't healthy. In our diets, protein is the main source of nitrogen, which is the predominant waste product eliminated by our kidneys. Excessive protein subjects us to too much nitrogen and puts an unneeded burden on our kidneys. Too little protein creates weak muscles, fatigue, mental lethargy, and, eventually, poor immune function. A happy medium is to eat a combination of daily broth, which contains valuable essential amino acids, 1–2 eggs per day, and flesh food (meat, organ meats, fish, poultry). The portion of the latter should be about the size of a deck of cards per day, although for large people, especially males, it can be doubled to a portion the size of a deck of cards twice per day. That said, it's a good dietary practice to not overeat protein at one sitting and to limit the amount of pure protein food to this deck-of-cards size per meal.

Principle Five: Water

There have been hundreds, maybe thousands of different diet books written in the past few decades. Yet, almost without exception, none of them mention, even in passing, the type of water their readers should drink or use in cooking. Yet water is the single largest "food" substance we ingest. And modern water purification methods, while making our municipal tap water safe bacteriologically, leave chemical residues, which are unsafe to ingest even at low concentrations. The two most common examples of these toxic additives in most municipal water supplies are chloramines, the form of chloride used to sterilize the water, and fluoride, a toxic enzyme inhibitor.[3] This is not going to be a treatise on the toxicity of fluoride or chloramines in water because you can easily find information about that on the Internet. And these are not the only toxic substances found in most municipal water supplies. Studies have shown that most municipal water contains relevant amounts of pharmaceutical drugs, metals, and the chemicals used in the production of sunscreens.[4] For these reasons, I'm including some instructions on how to treat your own water supply to avoid exposure.

There's another aspect of our drinking water that we need to consider, based on the research of Viktor Schauberger and simple common sense. Many of us intuitively sense that water is not the dead, inert vehicle it is made out to be. Fresh, moving water or water bubbling out of a spring has an elusive life quality that defies chemical analysis but can be perceived by any reasonably sensitive person. Healthy water, or what Schauberger called "mature water," is cool and moves in spiral or vortex patterns. Overheated, stagnant water is a breeding ground for disease and, as any hiker knows, should be avoided.

So, first we need to remove the toxic "stuff" from the water, while leaving the healthy minerals and salts. Distilled water is not the answer, since this water is stripped of all the beneficial minerals that are dissolved in the water. And second, we need to make sure the water is cool and moving—in a spiral motion that mimics the spiraling movements of the heart. The goal, then, is to provide an abundant source of mineral-rich, toxin-free, cool, spiraling water. Apart from living near a remote mountain spring, this is a vexing problem, as currently there is no simple strategy available to the homeowner to provide such water. Furthermore, the systems I have heard of that most closely approximate what would be needed to produce such water are often prohibitively expensive for most people.

I know people and companies who are directly involved with working on this problem and coming up with effective solutions, and I welcome these developments, but there is no ready solution at this time. For now, I can only offer the strategy I use in my own home, although I realize it's not the ideal solution and involves controversial processes.

I get rid of the "stuff" with an under-the-sink kitchen Nikken filter. This is a multistage filtration device that removes most contaminants except fluoride. To remove the fluoride, I put one teaspoon of Adya Clarity mineral solution in a gallon jar of water and let it sit for 24–48 hours. Independent laboratory analysis has shown that the ionic minerals in the Adya Clarity bind to toxins including fluoride, causing them to precipitate and therefore be easily filtered out. After this 24–48 hour period, I put the precipitated water through a simple carbon filter that removes the precipitated matter from the water. Then I put this cleaner water in a vortex machine (called a Duet Water Revitalizer), which remineralizes the water and puts it into a vortex motion for nine minutes. I then store water in Flaska bottles in our refrigerator. For the most current information on the nature of water and how you can best treat your own water, consult the website www.dancingwithwater.com.

Principle Six:
Trust Your Instincts

Finally, we must acknowledge in a treatise on diet that eating is one of life's inherent joys. Any diet that takes the joy of eating away from you is suspect at best and dangerous at worst. Eating must remain a joyful and social experience, not a clinical and mechanical process, and everyone must ultimately find their own diet for themselves. I can give you principles based on my understanding of physiology and disease to guide you in making sound food choices, but ultimately you must carefully listen to and observe how you are reacting to the foods you are eating. One of the benefits I have seen over the years of putting people on this diet program is that by clarifying and simplifying their diets, many people do learn over time which diet is right for them. When you are eating the standard American diet, there is simply no strategy for distinguishing what is working from what is making you sick. By starting over, sticking to simple whole-some food, you will learn the lessons of how you need to eat. At that point, you become your own doctor, the wisdom of your own body becomes the guide, and you will be on the road to better health.

Sample Menus

Breakfast 1: One or two eggs prepared any way you like them. (Sautéed in coconut oil and topped with vegetable powders or mixed with an assortment of sautéed vegetables are particularly enjoyable ways to eat them.) Green tea with a teaspoon of coconut oil. One cup of fresh berries.

Breakfast 2: A large bowl of soup made from a bone broth base, a variety of sautéed vegetables, and a variety of sautéed natural sausages. Use coconut oil as the fat to sauté the vegetables and a combination of miso and natto to flavor the soup. Add a large spoonful of fermented vegetables to the top of the finished soup. Heart-friendly hibiscus tea with one teaspoon of coconut oil.

Lunch 1: A large salad with a variety of vegetables, including raw greens, lightly cooked and cooled vegetables (broccoli, cauliflower, kale, etc.), and cooked eggs, chicken, or fish (canned or fresh cooked). The salad dressing can be either olive oil and balsamic vinegar with a variety of herbs and spices or a salad dressing made from a beaten raw egg yolk and crème fraîche. Side dishes can include a variety of fermented vegetables, a small amount of raw milk cheese, berries, or apple slices.

Lunch 2: Poached salmon topped with butter, ghee, or coconut oil and herbs with a large serving of lightly steamed or sautéed vegetables in coconut oil, butter, or ghee. Rooibos tea with a teaspoon of coconut oil and fresh berries can finish the meal.

Dinner 1: A four- to six-ounce serving of protein (fish, meat, or poultry), a small serving of either sweet potato or gluten-free grain (e.g., brown rice or quinoa), and a large serving of a big variety of vegetables. For example, baked chicken with rice and stir-fried vegetables. Side dishes should include fermented vegetables and a cup of soup if you didn't have it already for breakfast.

Dinner 2: Slow-cooker stews are economical and efficient meals. A basic beef stew that substitutes sweet potato for white potato can be a family staple. To this, I would add a large green salad with a wide variety of cooked and raw vegetables. Then add a fermented vegetable, a cup of soup with vegetable powders, and a variety of berries or a few slices of tropical fruit for dessert.

On the fasting days, omit the breakfast meal and, if need be, push the lunch meal forward for a few hours.

Preventing and Treating Angina, Unstable Angina, and Heart Attacks

First, a caveat: Like all medical treatments, this is best carried out in conjunction with your cardiologist and a physician familiar with this therapy. There is no generic "patient," so there can be no generic treatment plan, so the best results will come from working together with your doctor and making adjustments. The following outline is where I start, adjusting from there.

1. Adjust your diet following the guidelines in appendix A until the hsCRP (for inflammation) and HgbA1c (for blood sugar control) are normal. The optimal A1c level is between

4.9 and 5.4, not the usual normal listed in the lab guidelines. The hsCRP should be always less than 1.0; less than 0.5 is better.

2. Emu oil such as from www.walkabouthealthproducts.com. The dose is three capsules twice per day.

3. *Strophanthus*. *Strophanthus* is currently hard to obtain in the United States. The most to least favorable options are:

   a. G-strophanthin (ouabain). Currently the only world-wide source is a compounding pharmacy in Germany that will make it up under a doctor's order. It comes in 3 mg capsules, and the starting dose is one capsule before meals twice per day. Adjust from there based on how you feel, the effect on stamina, chest pains (angina), heart rate, and stress echo results. The final dose is usually between 3 mg up to a maximum of 18 mg per day (this highest dose is rarely needed).

   b. *Strophanthus* extract. This is an extract of the *Strophanthus* plant itself, which contains g-strophanthin. The positive aspect of this medicine is that it contains all of the cofactors contained in the plant itself. As of this writing, the only currently available source of this extract is from an herbal company in Brazil called TeeBrasil (www.teebrasil.com). I have used this for many years with uniformly positive results. The directions are five to twenty drops of the extract in a small amount of water, held in the mouth for one minute before swallowing, three times per day before meals. Again, adjust the dose based on your reaction.

   c. Strophactiv D4. This is a German homeopathic product that is a D4 potency of g-strophanthin. It is very dilute and mild but still effective, especially for sensitive people. The rationale for using dilute doses is that g-strophanthin is an endogenous hormone, made in our own adrenal glands, that is also found in very dilute amounts in our blood. It is possible that the homeopathic amounts reflect our basic endogenous levels. This is also available without a prescription. The dose of strophactiv D4 is twenty drops in a teaspoon of water three times per day before meals, best held in your mouth for one minute before swallowing.

———◆———

To my knowledge, rarely have any of these *Strophanthus* preparations caused anyone any serious negative side effects. However, it is important, as with any medicine, to take only what is needed, to take it on a consistent basis, and to consult with your physician before using any form of *Strophanthus*.

Cholesterol and How to Read a Lipid Profile

I n approximately one of twenty my new patients, the main complaint is high cholesterol. They have been told to start statin drugs, and they are seeking a different opinion. This is an attempt to explain what you need to know if you are in that situation and to explain my understanding of the role (if any) that cholesterol has in the prevention or treatment of heart disease.

Up until about ten years ago, the theory of the cause of plaque development (and hence heart disease) was that there are various types of fats bound to protein floating around in our blood. The two most important for heart disease development are LDL (low-density lipoprotein) and HDL (high-density lipoprotein). LDL is considered the "bad" guy in this play because it delivers atherogenic (plaque-causing) substances to the arteries, thereby leading to their deposition. HDL, on the other hand, is the "good" guy because it picks up these atherogenic fats and carries them away from the arteries back to the liver to be metabolized. The whole of preventative cardiology and low-fat diet therapy is about decreasing LDL and increasing HDL.

Statins and low-fat diets work by lowering the LDL and, if you combine that with exercise, you have the Ornish and Pritikin Programs for the reversal of heart disease. When you take a lipid profile, you are measuring the total cholesterol, the triglycerides (another type of fat in the body, which is mostly the storage form of carbohydrates), the LDL, and the HDL. For years, the most sensitive indicator of cardiovascular risk has been considered the cholesterol/HDL ratio, and 3.5 was the magic number. Anything below 3.5 and the risk of heart disease was minimal.

Recently, however, cardiologists are putting more stock in the absolute level of the LDL. While there are different opinions on the optimal value of LDL, most are saying the lower the better.[1] Modern cardiology routinely aims for LDL levels below 100 or even below 80 if there is a prior history of heart disease. It is also worth noting that the triglycerides are inversely related to the "protective" HDL so that, when the triglycerides go up (usually from excess carbohydrate exposure or sometimes alcohol consumption), the HDLs will go down.[2] To summarize then, from a conventional cardiology perspective, you want a cholesterol/HDL ratio of less than 3.5 and an LDL of less than 100 or, if you have had prior heart disease, less than 80. That is the company line.

However, two published articles have a different take. The first paper, published in the *British Medical Journal* in 2000, was a twenty-year retrospective on the use of statin drugs in the treatment and prevention of heart disease.[3] The study's conclusion was that the benefit of statin drug therapy is mild, about a 7 percent to 10 percent risk reduction. (By the way, "risk reduction" is a clever way to manipulate data and thereby people. For example, take two groups of 500 patients each; in one group, you give Drug X and find that one person dies of a heart attack. In the placebo group, you give nothing and two people die of heart attacks. Risk reduction concludes that there is a 33 percent reduction in risk if you take Drug X. So you can't really put a lot of stock in the term.) Its other major conclusion was that while there was a modest (and perhaps meaningless) reduction in risk of heart disease, the overall all-cause mortality (meaning death from all causes) was unchanged as a result of statin use. In other words, statin use does not change the possibility of dying, it only creates a modest, and possibly suspect, reduction in the risk of heart disease.

In 2004, an expert in lipids named Uffe Ravnskov wrote an article for *Wise Traditions* called "The Benefits of High Cholesterol."[4] Dr. Ravnskov makes the case that LDL is largely responsible for preventing infections and that people with the lowest LDL levels have the highest overall mortality rate. Patients below 100 are the most at risk for death based on all-cause death rates (death from any cause, not just heart disease). He lays out a case that attempting to lower LDL should be rarely, if ever, undertaken.

I counsel my patients that the lipid profile is a highly questionable tool for assessing their risk of heart disease and that, if their cholesterol/HDL ratio is less than 3.5 (or close to 3.5), no intervention is needed or useful. Lastly, if their ratio is higher than 5.5 (usually because of high triglycerides and low HDL), they stand to benefit substantially from the guidelines in appendix A, including a low-carbohydrate diet to lower the triglyceride level, as well as a more active exercise program. Apart from that, there is little else of value that can be learned from this test, in my opinion.

NOTES

Chapter Two: Circulation

1. Robert A. Freitas Jr., *Nanomedicine, Volume I: Basic Capabilities* (Georgetown, TX: Landes Bioscience, 1999).
2. Gerald H. Pollack, *The Fourth Phase of Water* (Seattle, WA: Ebner and Sons Publishers, 2013).
3. Ibid., 82.
4. Ibid., 53.
5. Viktor Schauberger, *Nature as Teacher: New Principles in the Working of Nature (Ecotechnology)* (Dublin, Ireland: Gill Books, 1999).
6. Ibid.
7. Viktor Schauberger, *Living Water* (Dublin, Ireland: Gill & MacMillan, 2002), 22.
8. University of Leicester, "Breakthrough Discovery Reveals How Thirsty Trees Pull Water to Their Canopies," *ScienceDaily*, January 20, 2016, https://www.sciencedaily.com/releases/2016/01/160120092649.htm.

Chapter Three:
The Misery Index

1. "Misery Index (Economics)," *Wikipedia*, https://en.wikipedia.org/wiki/Misery_index_(economics).
2. World Health Organization, *Mental Health: A Call for Action by World Health Ministers* (World Health Organization, 2001), http://www.who.int/mental_health/advocacy/en/Call_for_Action_MoH_Intro.pdf.
3. Brandon H. Hidaka, "Depression as a Disease of Modernity: Explanations for Increasing Prevalence," *Journal of Affective Disorders* 140, no. 3 (November 2012): 205–214, http://www.ncbi.nlm.nih.gov/pubmed/22244375.
4. Donald A. Grinde Jr. and Bruce E. Johansen, *Exemplar of Liberty: Native America and the Evolution of Democracy* (American Indian Studies Center, UCLA, 1991).
5. Rudolf Steiner, *Course for Young Doctors* (Spring Valley, NY: Mercury Press, 1994).
6. Weston A. Price, *Nutrition and Physical Degeneration*, ed. Price-Pottenger Nutrition (Lemon Grove, CA: Price Pottenger Nutrition, 2009).

Chapter Four:
The Geometry of the Heart

1. Armin Husemann, *The Harmony of the Human Body* (Edinburgh, UK: Floris Books, 2003).
2. L. F. C. Mees, *Secrets of the Skeleton* (Great Barrington, MA: Steiner Books, 1995).
3. Seth Miller, *A New Sacred Geometry* (Spirit Alchemy Design, 2013), 12.
4. Ibid.

5. Frank Chester, "Home," *New Form Technology*, http://
www.frankchester.com.
6. Ibid., 3, 13.
7. Ibid., 13.

Chapter Six:
What Doesn't Cause Heart Attacks

1. "About Underlying Cause of Death, 1999–2014," Centers
for Disease Control and Prevention, accessed February 3,
2015, http://wonder.cdc.gov/ucd-icd10.html.
2. Giorgio Baroldi and Malcolm Silver, *The Etiopathogenesis of
Coronary Heart Disease: A Heretical Theory Based on
Morphology* (Texas: Landes Bioscience, 2004), http://www
.strophantus.de/mediapool/59/596780/data/Baroldi
_Heretical_2004.pdf; and Knut Sroka, "On the Genesis of
Myocardial Ischemia," *Z Kardiol* 93 (2004): 768–783,
http://heartattacknew.com/wp-content/uploads/2012
/12/on_the_genesis_of_myocardial_ischemia.pdf. I am
also indebted to the work of Dr. Knut Sroka and his
website, www.heartattacknew.com.
3. "Heart Disease Facts," Centers for Disease Control and
Prevention, accessed May 26, 2016, http://www.cdc.gov
/heartdisease/facts.htm.
4. "Heart Disease and Stroke Cost America Nearly $1 Billion
a Day in Medical Costs, Lost Productivity," CDC
Foundation, April 29, 2015, http://www.cdcfoundation
.org/pr/2015/heart-disease-and-stroke-cost-america
-nearly-1-billion-day-medical-costs-lost-productivity.
5. C. S. Rihal et al., "Indications for Coronary Artery Bypass
Surgery and Percutaneous Coronary Intervention in
Chronic Stable Angina," *Circulation* 108, no. 20
(November 2003): 2439–2445, http://www.ncbi.nlm.nih
.gov/pubmed/14623791.

6. Knut Sroka, "The Riddle's Solution," Heart Attack New Approaches, http://heartattacknew.com/faq/how -dangerous-are-my-blocked-coronary-arteries/the -riddles-solution.

7. Pam Belluck, "Cholesterol-Fighting Drugs Show Wider Benefit," *New York Times*, November 9, 2008, http://www .nytimes.com/2008/11/10/health/10heart.html.

8. W. Doerr, W. W. Höpker, and J. A. Roßner, *Neues und Kritisches vom und zum Herzinfarkt: Vorgelegt in der Sitzung vom 14. Dezember 1974 (Sitzungsberichte der Heidelberger Akademie der Wissenschaften)* (Springer, 1975).

9. Giorgio Baroldi and Malcolm Silver, *The Etiopathogenesis of Coronary Heart Disease: A Heretical Theory Based on Morphology* (Texas: Landes Bioscience, 2004).

10. R. H. Helfant et al., "Coronary Heart Disease. Differential Hemodynamic, Metabolic and Electrocardiographic Effects in Subjects with and without Angina during Atrial Pacing," *Circulation* 42, no. 4 (October 1970): 601–610, http:// www.ncbi.nlm.nih.gov/pubmed/11993303.

Chapter Seven:
What Does Cause Heart Attacks

1. Giorgio Baroldi and Malcolm Silver, *The Etiopathogenesis of Coronary Heart Disease: A Heretical Theory Based on Morphology* (Texas: Landes Bioscience, 2004), http://www .strophantus.de/mediapool/59/596780/data/Baroldi _Heretical_2004.pdf; Knut Sroka, "On the Genesis of Myocardial Ischemia," *Z Kardiol* 93 (2004): 768–783, http://heartattacknew.com/wp-content/uploads/2012 /12/on_the_genesis_of_myocardial_ischemia.pdf; H. Fürstenwerth, "Ouabain—the Insulin of the Heart," *The International Journal of Clinical Practice* 64, no. 12 (November 2010): 1591–1594, http://www

.herzinfarkt-alternativen.de/wp-content/uploads/2012/12
/ouabain_the_insulin_of_the_heart.pdf; and H.
Fürstenwerth, "On the Differences between Ouabain and
Digitalis Glycosides," *American Journal of Therapeutics* 21,
no. 1 (January–February 2014): 35–42, http://www.ncbi
.nlm.nih.gov/pubmed/21642827.

2. Knut Sroka, "On the Genesis of Myocardial Ischemia," *Z
Kardiol* 93 (2004): 768–783, http://heartattacknew.com
/wp-content/uploads/2012/12/on_the_genesis_of
_myocardial_ischemia.pdf.

3. B. Takase et al., "Heart Rate Variability in Patients with
Diabetes Mellitus, Ischemic Heart Disease and Congestive
Heart Failure," *Journal of Electrocardiology* 25, no. 2 (April
1992): 79–88, http://www.ncbi.nlm.nih.gov/pubmed
/1522401.

4. Knut Sroka, "On the Genesis of Myocardial Ischemia," *Z
Kardiol* 93 (2004): 768–783, http://heartattacknew.com
/wp-content/uploads/2012/12/on_the_genesis_of
_myocardial_ischemia.pdf.

5. Knut Sroka et al., "Heart Rate Variability in Myocardial
Ischemia during Daily Life," *Journal of Electrocardiology* 30,
no. 1 (January 1997): 45–56, http://www.ncbi.nlm.nih
.gov/pubmed/9005886.

6. Knut Sroka, "On the Genesis of Myocardial Ischemia," *Z
Kardiol* 93 (2004): 768–783, http://heartattacknew.com
/wp-content/uploads/2012/12/on_the_genesis_of
_myocardial_ischemia.pdf.

7. James Scheuer and Norman Brachfeld, "Coronary
Insufficiency: Relations between Hemodynamic, Electrical,
and Biochemical Parameters," *Circulation Research* (1966):
178–189, http://circres.ahajournals.org/content/18/2
/178; and P. G. Schmid et al., "Regional Choline
Acetyltransferase Activity in the Guinea Pig Heart,"
Circulation Research (1978): 657–660, http://circres
.ahajournals.org/content/42/5/657.

8. A. M. Katz, "Effects of Ischemia on the Cardiac Contractile Proteins," *Cardiology* 56, no. 1 (1971): 276–283, http://www.ncbi.nlm.nih.gov/pubmed/4261989.

9. Weston A. Price, *Nutrition and Physical Degeneration* (Price Pottenger Nutrition, 2009).

10. Debra Braverman, *Heal Your Heart with EECP* (Celestial Arts, 2005).

11. Ibid.

Chapter Ten:
The Cosmic Heart

1. "The Top 10 Causes of Death," World Health Organization, updated May 2014, accessed May 26, 2016, http://www.who.int/mediacentre/factsheets/fs310/en.

2. Ta-Nehisi Coates, "Hoodlums," *The Atlantic*, December 7, 2010, http://www.theatlantic.com/national/archive/2010/12/hoodlums/67599.

3. Arild Vaktskjold et al., "The Mortality in Gaza in July–September 2014: A Retrospective Chart-Review Study," *Conflict and Health* 10, no. 10 (May 2016), http://www.ncbi.nlm.nih.gov/pmc/articles/PMC4855860.

4. "Science," *Merriam-Webster*, http://www.merriam-webster.com/dictionary/science.

5. Rollin McCraty et al., *The Coherent Heart* (California: Institute of HeartMath, 2006), http://www.heartmath.com/wp-content/uploads/2014/04/coherent_heart.pdf.

6. For example, John Hopkins Medicine puts normal adult respiration at 12–16 beats per minute. "Vital Signs (Body Temperature, Pulse Rate, Respiration Rate, Blood Pressure," *Johns Hopkins Medicine*, http://www.hopkinsmedicine.org/healthlibrary/conditions/cardiovascular_diseases/vital_signs_body_temperature_pulse_rate_respiration_rate_blood_pressure_85,P00866.

Chapter Eleven:
A Heart of Gold

1. Raj Chetty et al., "The Association between Income and Life Expectancy in the United States, 2001–2014," *Journal of the American Medical Association* 315, no. 16 (April 2016): 1750–1766, http://jama.jamanetwork.com /article.aspx?articleid=2513561.

2. James A. Levine, "Poverty and Obesity in the U.S.," *Diabetes* 60, no. 11 (November 2011): 2667–2668, http:// www.ncbi.nlm.nih.gov/pmc/articles/PMC3198075.

3. S. Saydah and K. Lochner, "Socioeconomic Status and Risk of Diabetes-Related Mortality in the U.S.," *Public Health Reports* 125, no. 3 (May–June 2010): 377–388, http:// www.ncbi.nlm.nih.gov/pubmed/20433032.

4. "Mental Health, Poverty and Development," World Health Organization, accessed May 26, 2016, http://www.who.int /mental_health/policy/development/en.

5. G. Lee and M. Carrington, "Tackling Heart Disease and Poverty," *Nursing Health & Science* 9, no. 4 (December 2007): 290–294, http://www.ncbi.nlm.nih.gov/pubmed /17958679.

6. "Poverty," *Merriam-Webster*, http://www.merriam-webster .com/dictionary/poverty.

7. Rakesh Kochhar, "What It Means to Be Poor by Global Standards," Pew Research Center, published July 22, 2015, http://www.pewresearch.org/fact-tank/2015/07/22/what -it-means-to-be-poor-by-global-standards; see also Rakesh Kochhar, "A Global Middle Class Is More Promise than Reality," Pew Research Center, July 8, 2015, http://www .pewglobal.org/2015/07/08/a-global-middle-class-is -more-promise-than-reality.

8. "Poverty Guidelines," U.S. Department of Health & Human Services, January 1, 2015, https://aspe.hhs.gov /poverty-guidelines.

9. Tim Henderson, "Poverty Rate Drops in 24 States, DC," PEW Charitable Trusts, September 18, 2015, http://www .pewtrusts.org/en/research-and-analysis/blogs/ stateline/2015/09/18/poverty-rate-drops-in-34-states-dc; "World Bank Forecasts Global Poverty to Fall Below 10% for First Time; Major Hurdles Remain in Goal to End Poverty by 2030," The World Bank, October 4, 2015, http://www.worldbank.org/en/news/press-release/2015 /10/04/world-bank-forecasts-global-poverty-to-fall-below -10-for-first-time-major-hurdles-remain-in-goal-to-end -poverty-by-2030; and "2. Background," World Health Organization, accessed May 26, 2016, http://www.who .int/nutrition/topics/2_background/en.

10. Raj Chetty et al., "The Association between Income and Life Expectancy in the United States, 2001–2014," *Journal of the American Medical Association* 315, no. 16 (2016): 1750–1766.

11. Ellen Brown, "Who Owns the Federal Reserve?," Global Research, September 30, 2015, http://www.globalresearch .ca/who-owns-the-federal-reserve/10489.

12. Bart Gruzalski, "The USA Attacked Iraq Because Saddam Had W$D," *Counterpunch*, March 22, 2013, http://www .counterpunch.org/2013/03/22/ the-usa-attacked-iraq-because-saddam-had-wd.

13. Brad Hoff, "Hillary Emails Reveal True Motive for Libya Intervention," *Foreign Policy Journal*, January 6, 2016, http://www.foreignpolicyjournal.com/2016/01/06 /new-hillary-emails-reveal-true-motive-for-libya -intervention.

Chapter Twelve:
What's Love Got to Do with It?

1. Paul Pearsall, *The Heart's Code* (Danvers, MA: Broadway Books, 1999), 88–90.

Appendix A:
The Cowan Heart Diet

1. G. Taormina and M.G. Mirisola, "Longevity: Epigenetic and Biomolecular Aspects," *Biomolecular Concepts* 6, no. 2 (Apr. 2015): 105–117, http://www.ncbi.nlm.nih.gov /pubmed/25883209.
2. K. C. Bedi Jr. et al., "Evidence for Intramyocardial Disruption of Lipid Metabolism and Increased Myocardial Ketone Utilization in Advanced Human Heart Failure," *Circulation* 133, no. 8 (Feb. 2016): 706–716, http://www .ncbi.nlm.nih.gov/pubmed/26819374.
3. Water Quality Association, "Common Waterborne Contaminants," *Water Quality Association*, https://www .wqa.org/learn-about-water/common-contaminants.
4. WHO, *Pharmaceuticals in Drinking-water* (Geneva, Switzerland: World Health Organization, 2011), http:// www.who.int/water_sanitation_health/publications/2011 /pharmaceuticals_20110601.pdf.

Appendix C:
Cholesterol and How to Read a Lipid Profile

1. M. Farnier, "Future Lipid-Altering Therapeutic Options Targeting Residual Cardiovascular Risk," *Current*

Cardiology Reports 18, no. 7 (July 2016): 65, http://www
.ncbi.nlm.nih.gov/pubmed/27216845.

2. W. Masson et al., "Association Between Triglyceride/HDL
Cholesterol Ratio and Carotid Atherosclerosis in
Postmenopausal Middle-Aged Women," *Endocrinología y
Nutrición* S1575-0922, no. 16 (May 2016): 30047–X,
http://www.ncbi.nlm.nih.gov/pubmed/27236636.

3. M. Pignone, C. Phillips, and C. Mulrow, "Use of Lipid
Lowering Drugs for Primary Prevention of Coronary Heart
Disease: Meta-analysis of Randomised Trials," *British
Medical Journal* 321, no. 7267 (October 2000): 983–986,
http://www.ncbi.nlm.nih.gov/pubmed/11039962.

4. Uffe Ravnskov, "The Benefits of High Cholesterol," The
Weston A. Price Foundation, June 24, 2004, http://www
.westonaprice.org/modern-diseases/the-benefits-of-high
-cholesterol/.

RECOMMENDED READING

Books

Anderson, M. Kat. *Tending the Wild: Native American Knowledge and the Management of California's Natural Resources*. Berkeley: University of California Press, 2006.

Cowan, Thomas, MD. *How (and Why) to Eat More Vegetables*. San Francisco, CA: Thomas Cowan, MD, 2016.

Cowan, Thomas, MD. *The Fourfold Path to Healing*. Washington, DC: New Trends Publishing, 2004.

Eisenstein, Charles. *Sacred Economics*. Berkeley, CA: Evolver Editions, 2011.

Eisenstein, Charles. *The More Beautiful World Our Hearts Know Is Possible*. Berkeley, CA: North Atlantic Books, 2013.

Fallon, Sally. *Nourishing Traditions*. Washington, DC: New Trends Publishing, 2000.

Illich, Ivan. *Deschooling Society*. New York: Harper and Row, 2000.

Illich, Ivan. *Medical Nemesis*. New York: Pantheon Books, 1976.

Illich, Ivan. *The Right to Useful Unemployment*. New York: Marion Boyars, 1978.

Jensen, Derrick. *Dreams*. New York: Seven Stories Press, 2011.

Kashtan, Miki. *Reweaving the Human Fabric: Working Together to Create a Nonviolent Future*. Oakland, CA: Fearless Heart Publications, 2014.

Miller, Seth. *A New Sacred Geometry: The Art and Science of Frank Chester*. Spirit Alchemy Design, 2013.

Pollack, Gerald H. *The Fourth Phase of Water*. Washington, DC: Ebner and Sons Publishers, 2013.

Price, Weston A. *Nutrition and Physical Degeneration*, edited by Price-Pottenger Nutrition. Lemon Grove, CA: Price-Pottenger Nutrition, 2009.

Ralph Marinelli, Branko Furst, Hoyte van der Zee, Andrew McGinn, and William Marinelli, "The Heart Is Not a Pump: A Refutation of the Pressure Propulsion Premise of Heart Function," *Frontier Perspectives* 5, no. 1 (Fall-Winter (1995): 15-24, http://www.rsarchive.org/RelArtic/Marinelli.

Stefanson, Vilhjalmur. *Cancer: A Disease of Civilization*. New York: Hill and Wang, 1960.

Websites

Chester, Frank. "Home." *New Form Technology*. http://www .frankchester.com.

Dancing With Water. http://www.dancingwithwater.com.

Heart Attack New. http://www.heartattacknew.com.

The Fearless Heart. http://thefearlessheart.org.

Walkabout Health Products (for emu oil). http://walkabout healthproducts.com.

TeeBrasil (for *Strophanthus* extract). http://www.teebrasil.com.

The Weston A. Price Foundation. http://www.westonaprice.org.

Dr. Cowan's Garden. https://www.drcowansgarden.com.

Dr. Cowan's Fourfold Healing. http://fourfoldhealing.com.

INDEX

abdomen, examination of, 79
acetylcholine, 57, 59, 103
acidosis, lactic acid, 58
Activator X, 62
Adya Clarity mineral solution, 130
agriculture, community-supported, 45, 67
amnesia in statin therapy, 76–77
amyotrophic lateral sclerosis, 103
angina, 48, 50, 75
   EECP technique in, 63, 83
   unstable, 48, 50, 63, 75
angiography of coronary arteries, 51–52
   artifacts in, 53
   vascular spasms in, 51, 53
angioplasty in coronary artery stenosis, 50
animals
   grass-fed, 62, 127, 128
   as protein source, 128–129
   quality of foods from, 122
annual vegetables, 124
anthroposophical medicine, 24, 25–26, 41–46, 65–66

antimony, 26
anvil theory of medicine, 76
aortic arch, 8
   in hydraulic ram model of heart, 39
   in systole, 39
aortic valve, 36, 39
apex of heart
   muscle layer at, 36, 37
   position of, 34
arteries
   blood flow in, 8, 9, 18
   hypertension in, 9
arterioles, 8
arteriosclerosis, 60, 62
   diet in, 62, 138
   in inflammation, 19–20, 62
   plaque in. *See* plaque
arthritis, 62, 125
Ashitaba, 124
aspirin, 55, 57, 76
atherosclerosis, 19–20, 138
atria, 23, 30, 37
   in hydraulic ram model of heart, 38, 39

ABOUT
THE AUTHOR

Thomas Cowan, MD, has studied and written about many subjects in medicine, including nutrition, homeopathy, anthroposophical medicine, and herbal medicine. He is the principal author of *The Fourfold Path to Healing* and coauthor (with Sally Fallon) of *The Nourishing Traditions Book of Baby and Childcare.*

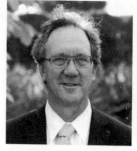

Ingrid Hatton Photography

Dr. Cowan has served as vice president of the Physicians' Association for Anthroposophic Medicine and is a founding board member of The Weston A. Price Foundation®. He also writes the "Ask the Doctor" column in *Wise Traditions in Food, Farming, and the Healing Arts* (The Weston A. Price Foundation's quarterly magazine) and has lectured throughout the United States and Canada. He has three grown children and currently practices medicine in San Francisco where he resides with his wife, Lynda Smith.

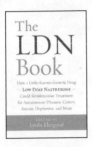
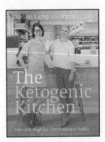
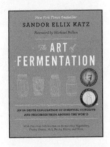
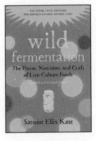
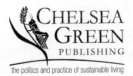

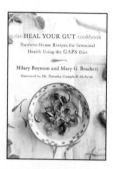
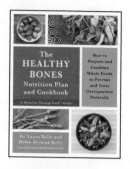
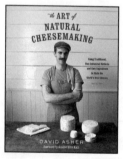
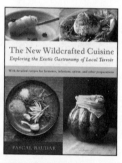
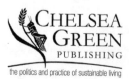